WOMB TO THRIVE

The Missing Keys to Heal Yourself, Your Family and the Planet

Compiled by Dr. Julie Gerland (*hc*)

Birthing The New Humanity

Disclaimer:
This book is written with the intention to create awareness, inspire, inform, and empower the reader with alternative methods that have worked for hundreds of women. However, the ideas, tools, philosophies should not be used as a substitute for the medical care you require.

If you are under medical or psychological supervision, you must consult your health care provider before using the information provided here.

Nothing in this book should be considered a guarantee of any results. Also, the ideas and philosophies shared in the book are not a substitute for proper medical or psychological care.

The publisher, designers, editors, contributors, and author shall not be liable for any loss or damage directly or indirectly because of the use or interpretation of any of the contents of the book.

Cover Design by Dr. François Gerland (*hc*), Gregory Moulinet & Shutterstock

Womb to Thrive, by Dr. Julie Gerland (*hc*)
ISBN: 9798800339314

"If we were to look after pregnant women,
in just fifty years, that's two generations,
we could close all our prisons
and all our hospitals."

– Omraam Mikhaël Aïvanhov

Acknowledgements

We would like to express our deepest gratitude for the ever-present sacred Light within all that exists.

Also, we give thanks for the guidance and support of the Great Masters of Humanity as they uplift our global family through this time of upheaval and awakening.

We honor the dedication and work of the co-authors of this book and all of the pioneers whose tireless work is contributing to changing the paradigm of early parenting and birth practices.

We are grateful to the countless doctors, midwives, healthcare professionals, and entrepreneurs who honor the sacredness of life and treat mothers, fathers, and their babies with the greatest respect, nurturing care, kindness, and honesty.

We wish to acknowledge the Birthing The New Humanity directors and team members for their inspiration, support, encouragement, and tireless contributions on all levels for conceiving, forming, and birthing this book and this movement.

Special thanks to Viki Winterton, her team, and all those who have assisted in birthing this anthology.

Lastly, we thank all future parents who prepare consciously in body, mind, and spirit to bring a soul into the world that can reach its full potential and thrive.

Table of Contents

Introduction

by Drs. Julie & François Gerland (*hc*)

"The world can't go on like this!" These words have echoed in the hallways of the United Nations and around the globe for decades in the midst of international conflict. Change is obviously needed. But questions of what we must do and how have led to endless debate and conflicts of interest. We need a lasting solution to our individual, societal, and global challenges. This book offers the missing keys and a chance to birth the change we wish for ourselves, our families, and our world.

In 1980, at the United Nations in New York, one of the world's foremost disarmament experts showed me the door when I said that world peace starts with the individual. He replied, astonished, "Are you trying to say that if I go home and beat my wife and kick my cat, that has something to do with world peace?" Upon leaving, I crossed the street, thinking, *If this "elite" individual doesn't understand that only peaceful people will create a peaceful world, conflict and violence will only continue to escalate.*

A few months later, I learnt something incredible that soon developed into my life's mission: we can prevent the tremendous suffering that leads to violent and destructive behavior by focusing on mothers. Many don't realize that mothers and their wombs can solve the global challenges that are costing us the earth, yet we know that herein lies the powerful solution to forming a world where our global human family can blossom in harmony with the natural world and our mother earth.

Contrary to popular belief, babies are not born with a clean slate. Not only are babies developing their brains and physical organs in the womb, but they are also conscious. Mothers really do form their baby's character, habits, strengths, and weaknesses from conception. Their delicate, vulnerable newborns have already completed their most formative months and downloaded the subconscious programs that will run their lives. The womb is undoubtedly the first environment that deserves our care and protection.

Decades later, armed with the solution and as the Chief UN Representative for an NGO on prenatal education, I attended as many UN events as possible with my husband François. Our team kept bringing attention to what seemed a most unlikely and surprising solution to achieving the Millennium Development Goals and then the Sustainable Development Goals. We presented a way to eradicate poverty and to achieve global health, peace, and the protection of the planet. Having discovered the prenatal origins of human suffering and the ensuing consequences, we eagerly shared this information wherever we could.

Years of intense inner work, meditation, and healing of our own prenatal and birth trauma, working with pregnant couples, learning from scientific pioneers, and attending global conferences confirmed what we had learnt from two great teachers.

Bulgarian masters Beinsa Douno and Omraam Mikhaël Aïvanhov have given in-depth teachings on the power mothers have during pregnancy. In 1939, Aïvanhov told a group of French doctors in Lyon that what mothers experience during pregnancy creates the inner core of their children. They were not ready to hear this message, and they chose to laugh at him. Decades later, science confirmed that it is not genes that determine our lives but rather epigenetic, or environmental, factors that trigger the expression of the genes. Our awareness of the womb being the baby's first environment is of crucial importance.

We both had the great fortune of meeting Omraam Mikhaël Aïvanhov more than forty years ago. We learnt that, during pregnancy, the mother not only forms the baby's physical body but also their emotional and mental faculties. Her thoughts, feelings, deep beliefs, as well as her environment all imprint on her unborn child. If she lives in fear and stress, the baby's long-term health, intelligence, and capacity for empathy and love will be compromised. In contrast, if mothers live happy, healthy, empowered pregnancies and are supported to spend time engaging with their unborn baby, the child feels wanted, loved, and cared for and develops a deep sense of belonging. Known as "attachment parenting," this is now hailed as a vital perspective for healthy development.

This knowledge has been presented by sages and ancient traditions for millennia. In the Vedas, sacred Hindu scriptures, this wisdom is known as Garbh Sanskar, or education in the womb. However, over time and within our patriarchal societies, this knowledge has been nearly completely lost. Only a few traces remain, which are often regarded as unscientific or superstitious. In 1982, Canadian psychiatrist Dr. Thomas Verny published his best-selling book, "The Secret Life of the Unborn Child," and contemporary science finally made its debut on the subject. We are honored to have Dr. Verny as a co-author in this book.

As hypnotherapists, we observe the buried but ever-present suffering that stems from the earliest moments of life. Following precise protocols, we've had great success healing unconscious trauma, changing destructive habits, and overcoming limitations. These healing methods need to become mainstream and available to all. We now teach people how to access their own inner resources and make updates to their programs, just as one does for their computer. **It's not rocket science, it's neuroscience!**

Our convictions were strengthened when we met a British psychiatrist who had been commissioned by the government to investigate in high-security prisons and find out how murderers and high-level sex offenders become so violent. He confidentially revealed his findings, telling us that such heinous crimes could be prevented in the future. His report suggested that both parents, from the beginning of pregnancy, take two years' leave from their work, with full salaries, to offer their child the best possible start in life. Attending parenting classes would be compulsory too. Parents would learn how to stop the intergenerational transmission of fear and violence. This, he said, would eliminate tremendous suffering and be much more effective and cheaper than running costly prisons.

We continued our lobbying by organizing an event at the United Nations Earth Summit Rio+20 in 2012. With our partner organizations and global birth pioneer Dr. Michel Odent, we offered the only effective long-term solution: If human beings were given the best start in life from conception, through pregnancy, birth, and infancy, they would grow up healthy and loving and naturally create a paradise on earth for all.

Our lobbying bore fruit when, in 2018, unable to ignore the growing body of scientific literature, UN agencies including UNICEF produced a ground-breaking document: *Nurturing Care for Early Childhood Development: A framework for helping children survive and thrive to transform health and human potential.* It read, "During pregnancy and the first three years after birth, we lay down the critical elements of our health, well-being, and productivity, which will last throughout childhood, adolescence, and adulthood."

This book is a wakeup call for humanity. Far from the fear mongering noise of mainstream media, digital marketplaces, and town halls, this mighty new light is dawning on humanity. A global revolution is now taking place: Global peace, happiness, prosperity, and health will never come from politicians, academics, or corporations, as they do not hold the keys to a thriving world.

Mothers hold these keys!

Unfortunately, mothers are often routinely ignored, pushed out, undervalued, mistreated, violated, and traumatized. Many don't even have a say in how and where they will birth their babies, and in the 21st century, suicide is still the leading cause of death for pregnant women. Devoid of social status and excluded from the elaboration of policies and the education that influence and mould their children, mothers end up passing on to their children the stress, anguish, and frustration they endure.

In this critically important time of early development, birth holds special importance. Yet, according to research scientist Dr. Rachel Reed, "Obstetric violence is on the rise, and one in every three women are traumatized during childbirth."

Birth is still shrouded in fear, stress, ignorance, drama, domination, and mystery. It has received a lot of bad press and is often portrayed as dramatic, painful, and necessarily medically assisted. Having learnt from pioneer Marie Mongan, founder of the HypnoBirthing method, and then teaching this knowledge to parents and trained professionals for over two decades, we know that nothing is further from the truth.

The toxic cocktail of stress and fear hormones interferes with women's natural ability to birth comfortably. Birth was never meant to be the painful humiliating ordeal many mothers, fathers, and babies experience today. When mothers feel safe, loved, and supported, they naturally secrete oxytocin, the love hormone active during childbirth. Then, birth resembles a beautiful dance and becomes a celebration of life in love and joy. It's time for women to reclaim their birthing rights, swapping the medical business and profiteering hijackers for real love and the support of professional midwives and doulas. Medical intervention should only happen when strictly necessary.

Like the ever-changing cycles of nature, the tides are turning. The great Mother of humanity is awakening in the collective consciousness. Woman is and will always be the mother of man. She has been endowed with the instinct and intuition to know what is best for her children and to provide optimal conditions for their development. When she is disempowered and her voice is silenced, her children, fed with stress, frustration, and anguish, become dysfunctional.

The chapters in this book are a testimonial to the great rebirth that is inevitably taking place. The co-authors are leading-edge doctors, midwives, psychologists, therapists, experts, and parents from around the globe. They are among the courageous pioneers whose dedication and perseverance lead this essential collective paradigm shift.

Finally, we'd like to point out that this book doesn't take any "side" in the pro-life, pro-choice debate. On the contrary, we seek to enlighten, add love, and express empathy for *all* human beings. Our aim is to uncover and heal the underlying causes of widespread fear, violence, and suffering that lead to destructive behavior. The time is *now* to embark collectively on this grandiose mission, the most important of all: to enlighten, protect, support, and empower mothers in the tremendous influence they have on their child in the womb.

Chapter 1

WELCOME: DISCOVERY TRAUMA AND RECOVERY

By Cherionna Menzam-Sills

My Story

I was one of those children that never felt like I belonged. I would have believed I'd been adopted if I hadn't looked so much like my family. My understanding of why I felt that way came years later through deep therapy and study of pre- and perinatal psychology.

I decided early on to become an Occupational Therapist (OT), drawing inspiration from an OT I worked with as a teenager in a nursing home. Although I later enjoyed aspects of OT hospital work, I suffered a concussion during a folk-dance workshop that turned my life around less than two years after graduating.

Landing on the back of my head on the hard concrete floor left me stunned, basically paralysed, for a short time. Once I could move, my friends escorted me to a mat at the side of the room so they could continue dancing. As I lay there, I turned my head and was touched to see a newborn baby on the mat next to mine, her parents having safely placed her there while they danced. When I look back, I realise the symbolic nature of this experience for me. I truly began a new life in that moment.

Although I was diagnosed with a mild concussion, persistent problems led me to seek care from a neurologist a year later. Another shock came when a brain scan revealed a deteriorative disease similar to multiple sclerosis (MS). Having worked with people with MS in hospital, I was familiar with its associated severe disability. After leaving the neurologist's office in a daze, something guided me not to follow through with the doctor's recommended spinal tap and instead to think of myself as healthy. I had never heard such advice and knew nothing of the power of the mind, but I soon learned more. Listening to an inner wisdom became my new way of life. My intuition led me to holistic healing methods, some of which I trained in and began to practice.

In the early '90s during my work as a bodyworker, I had two clients "birth" themselves off my treatment table. They were both big men, about a foot taller than me, but I managed to support them in following their urges to slide off the table onto the floor. These experiences profoundly affected both my clients and me. I found myself following my intuition to move to Boulder, Colorado, to study Dance/Movement Psychotherapy at a Buddhist-inspired school called Naropa. Here I was introduced to pre- and perinatal psychology. My passion was kindled through participation in a workshop with pre- and perinatal therapy pioneer William R. Emerson and other classes. I realised that this was my life calling, and I needed to continue my studies.

I spent the next five years pursuing my doctorate in pre- and perinatal psychology. Following William's advice, I had asked Jeane Rhodes to be on my MA thesis committee, as she had also investigated pre- and perinatal themes in movement in her research. Jeane then became the first person I believe to attain a PhD in pre- and perinatal psychology. Following her lead, I became the second. This supported me teaching at both Naropa and the Santa Barbara Graduate Institute, which had opened just as I graduated. Now, following six years of intensive study with William, I moved to Santa Barbara, where I worked intensively with another pre- and perinatal therapy pioneer, Raymond Castellino. I also studied Craniosacral Biodynamics and the mindful movement practice of Continuum, both involving fluid states of receptivity, reminiscent of the embryo.

After ten years of intensive study and healing, I experienced myself differently. I no longer worried about having MS. My physical health had dramatically improved, and I could see my health issues relating to the extreme toxicity I marinated in prenatally. I gestated in Sarnia, a town known as having the highest particulate levels in Canada, where my father worked at one of the several petrochemical plants. I also encountered my prenatal experience of my mother's ambivalence about being pregnant with me. Although she wanted children, she could not fully celebrate being pregnant, due to her discomfort with gaining weight, low self-esteem, and a difficult relationship with my father. Feeling and acknowledging my very early history liberated me from its hold, eventually facilitating a stable intimate relationship and home, which both had been previously unreachable for me. I finally felt like I belonged.

Discovery

Through my personal work with William and Ray, I became aware of important prenatal developmental milestones. *Discovery* is one that challenged many of us. William defined discovery as when the pregnancy is confirmed by a pregnancy test. This is usually around three weeks after conception. Although modern technology can confirm pregnancy earlier and some people know the moment they conceive, this point is often when the woman realises she has missed her period and takes the test.

How parents react to the news of pregnancy can deeply affect both their lives and their baby's. Parents may be thrilled but may also feel stressed, overwhelmed, hopeless, angry, confused, afraid, or not ready. I have worked with so many new mothers who had just wanted to take that one trip to India, finish their education, or establish more financial, professional, or relational stability before starting a family. Others, like my mother, consciously delight in being pregnant but harbour unconscious ambivalence, to which baby subconsciously responds.

Many conceptions are not planned (1). I often heard William declare that anything other than celebration at discovery is shocking for the baby. This event initiates a conscious relationship, hopefully a bonding relationship, between parents and child. The baby, being a highly sentient being, senses and responds to the parents' welcome or rejection. For example, I felt unsafe and rejected by my mother's ambivalence.

If you question that a tiny embryo whose brain has not even formed could be aware of parental attitudes, picture the little one as composed of cells. Cells, like unicellular organisms, perceive and react to their environment. At a basic level, they sense nourishment and toxicity – they are open to receive nourishment and contract and withdraw as protection from toxicity. Babies in the womb do the same. They sense the biochemical environment within their mother as well as the bio-energetic fields produced by her organs, tissues, and environment. In my case, this included my father's frequent rages and violence.

When a mother experiences shock, stress, fear, joy, anger, love, or other emotions, her internal biochemical environment expresses them. As scientist Candace Pert describes in her seminal book, *Molecules of Emotion,* our emotions affect our physical bodies. The emotional response to discovery of a pregnancy tends to be intense. It is one of those moments parents rarely forget. Babies also remember.

Remembering Discovery

Memories of prenatal experience, including discovery, are generally not *explicit* (conscious) but *implicit* (unconscious), and nonverbal memories can pervade our lives and relationships. Lacking conscious memory, we tend to unconsciously act out our history. Individuals not welcomed at discovery can repeatedly experience rejection in relationships, often accompanied by a sense of shame, of being inherently wrong or bad, and of not belonging.

Unplanned pregnancies may be unwanted or just come at a different time than the parents intended. Parents who wanted a child but are surprised by the timing often get over their initial feelings and can then welcome their child. This can have a reparative effect, facilitated by parents speaking to the baby (yes, even in the womb), letting their child know they are sorry they weren't ready to celebrate when they found out, and how excited they are now to welcome them.

Babies who are unwanted usually do not experience the benefit of parents changing their minds. The initial shock may be exacerbated by parental thoughts of or attempts at abortion or adoption planning. Both options can be terrifying for the little one, who is completely dependent on the mother for survival. Unintended pregnancy is unfortunately associated with higher rates of child abuse by both parents (2). This reflects stress for both the baby and the parents at discovery, marking a crucial initiation of their relationship.

Pre- and perinatal therapists often encounter the effects of discovery trauma. I have seen many clients having to unlearn the tendency to stay small and invisible, which they developed to avoid being discovered. As little ones, they expected rejection at discovery and tried to prevent this by hiding. I frequently see this in new therapists I supervise who have trouble letting prospective clients recognize that they exist. They feel unable to create a website or business card, as if their fear of being discovered is still freezing their ability to act.

In relationships, people with discovery trauma may also stay small, avoiding asserting themselves with their partner, boss, neighbours, etc. They may struggle with commitment for fear of being rejected again. Have you ever had the thought, "If they ever found out who I really am, they would reject me"? This fear often presents physically as a collapsed chest, like being curled up in protection. Alternatively, this tendency may be overridden by stiffly holding the chest out in military fashion.

The Heart of the Matter

The physical remnants of discovery trauma can go beyond habitual posture. On a practical level, unintended pregnancies may take longer to be discovered and are associated with less prenatal care, lower rates of breastfeeding, and lower birth weight, all of which can affect the child's health (3). Significantly, the time of discovery usually corresponds to the heart beginning to beat.

The heart is the first organ to come online in an embryo. It begins as blood vessels forming at the head end of the embryo, known as the cardiogenic (heart-generating) region. The developing ectoderm, which develops primarily into the brain and nervous system, grows faster than other embryonic tissues and begins to expand over the developing heart. During the third week, the embryo appears to fold, bringing the heart to the centre, where it seemingly miraculously begins to beat. This is when discovery usually happens.

In development, body regions most actively changing tend to be most affected by events occurring at the time. Implicit memories of trauma or shock associated with being rejected at discovery are often stored in the heart or chest area, which tends to be collapsed and hold intense feelings. The heart can carry tender emotions of grief at the loss of potential connection with the parents, fear or terror of being annihilated, or suppressed love that could never be shared. Experiences of loss, rejection, abandonment, or other traumas can reinforce these very early discovery emotions. Is it any wonder that people with discovery trauma focus on avoiding rejection and loss in their relationships? They also might have trouble breathing, tending to hold their breath as if they were still in the moment of being discovered.

Healing, Recovery, and Prevention

Fortunately, these issues, along with other very early challenging influences, can be addressed in healing ways and can be prevented through awareness. Parents-to-be benefit from pre-conception support to work through their own early history and prevent re-enacting it in their relationships. Those who have experienced prenatal rejection often unconsciously recreate this with their own children. For example, a woman who felt unwanted at her own discovery might unconsciously conceive and have an abortion at the same age her mother was at her own conception. Therapy can help bring these experiences to awareness, supporting the woman to conceive consciously when she is ready to truly welcome the little one she is bringing into the world. If an unconscious conception has occurred earlier, with abortion or adoption following, therapy can also help the woman to process her feelings, enabling her to later welcome a child with clarity when the time is right. Prenatal therapy can also help heal such very early wounding, facilitating stable, loving, intimate relationships that can sincerely welcome a baby into the family.

If unintended pregnancy does occur, parents need support to work through their feelings and find ways to make repair with their baby, as suggested earlier. This can happen before or after birth, but earlier repair reduces how long the child suffers. If you are a parent of an older child, please do not despair! Repair is possible at any time. Please also have compassion for yourself. You did what you knew how and were able to do at the time. If you can forgive yourself and express your regrets and apology to your child, you will be amazed at the results.

Pre- and perinatal therapy can support children of any age to recover from very early trauma, like being rejected at discovery. Within the safe, supportive relational field of therapy, change can happen at a cellular level. Cells that withdrew from the sense of danger back then can open and expand again as they sense safety. If you experienced less than celebration at discovery, it is never too late to celebrate yourself. You might consider the very tiny one you were back then, heart just beginning to beat. Remembering your current age and all you are capable of now as an adult, what might you want to offer that little being you once were? Often, that embryo just needs to be welcomed. Can you welcome that little you? Notice what you sense in your body, your breath, and your heart as you do this.

Welcome is a first principle in the somatic pre- and perinatal therapy I learned from Ray Castellino. In the small womb surround process workshops and classes I offer, we begin with welcome. Where discovery was not welcoming, a new experience is possible. We can even practice discovering and welcoming each moment. What might be available for *you* to discover and welcome in this moment? As we heal in this way, we more easily meet ourselves and each other with compassion, supporting gentler births and a more peaceful, cooperative, compassionate world.

References

1. Bearak, J., Popinchalk, A., Alkema, L., and Sedgh, G. (2018). "Global, regional, and subregional trends in unintended pregnancy and its outcomes from 1990 to 2014: estimates from a Bayesian hierarchical model". *The Lancet. Global Health.* **6** (4): e380–e389. doi:10.1016/S2214-109X(18)30029-9. PMC 6055480. PMID 29519649.

2. Guterman, K., (2015). Unintended pregnancy as a predictor of child maltreatment, *Child Abuse & Neglect, 48*: 160-169, ISSN 0145-2134, https://doi.org/10.1016/j.chiabu.2015.05.014. (https://www.sciencedirect.com/science/article/pii/S014

5213415001945)

3. Kost, K. and Lindberg, L. (2015). Pregnancy Intentions, Maternal Behaviors, and Infant Health: Investigating Relationships With New Measures and Propensity Score Analysis, *Demography, 52* (1): 83–111. https://doi.org/10.1007/s13524-014-0359-9

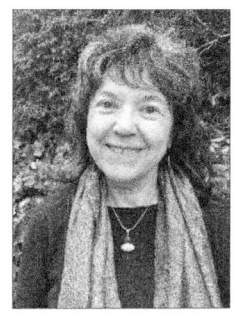 **Cherionna Menzam-Sills** has been a somatic prenatal and birth therapist and Craniosacral therapist since the '90s. Informed by her PhD in Pre- and Perinatal Psychology (PPN) and extensive study with PPN pioneers, William Emerson and Ray Castellino, she has taught PPN, Embodied Embryology, Continuum, a mindful movement practice, and Biodynamic Craniosacral Therapy globally. She has also authored two books, *The Breath of Life: An Introduction to Craniosacral Biodynamics* and *Spirit into Form: Exploring Embryological Potential and Prenatal Psychology.*

Chapter 2

HOW I DISCOVERED PRE- AND PERI-NATAL PSYCHOLOGY

By Thomas R. Verny, MD

Looking back many years, I think this is how my interest in early memories were awakened. One day, while working with a young man on his dream, he suddenly started to cry, without any input from me. He cried for close to ten minutes and then stopped on his own. "What did you just experience?" I asked him. He told me that, in his mind, he found himself in a crib and that he was crying for his mother. Then, he recalled that he had actually seen photos of himself as an infant and some of them pictured him lying in a blue crib whereas the crib that he had just experienced was definitely white. He wondered about the discrepancy. I suggested that he ask his mother for more information.

The next week he returned for his regular appointment and told me that, according to his mother, when he was born, his parents lacked money for a new crib but were able to borrow one from a neighbor. The borrowed crib was white. A few months later, they could afford to buy a new crib for him, and that new crib was blue. That is the one that appears in all of the early photographs.

I felt both intrigued and mystified by this experience, since throughout my studies, first at the University of Toronto then Harvard University I was taught that children remember nothing before the age of two. Yet, as I continued to practice psychiatry,

I repeatedly encountered patients who would tell me about events in their lives that reached far back in time to infancy, birth, and even womb life. A few of these memories may have originated from overheard conversations by family members or gleaned from photo albums or videos.

On the other hand, a considerable number would not have been easily available and were corroborated by evidence supplied by parents, hospital reports, and other documentation. I wondered how to explain these memories scientifically. After considerable study, I submitted a paper "The Psychic Life of the Unborn Child" to the 5th World Congress of Psychosomatic Obstetrics and Gynecology Rome, Italy, Nov. 1977.

To my great surprise, my paper was accepted. Even more surprisingly, I was given prime time to present it. My paper was so well received that, at the end of my talk, I suggested that if anyone wanted to continue the conversation, please come to my room at 5 pm.

At the appointed time, people were lining up to get into my room. There was much excitement. I met R. D. Laing, Sheila Kitzinger, Frederick Leboyer, Louis Mehl, and Susanne Arms, among many others. It became very apparent to me that this was a subject that was of immense interest to some of the brightest, most accomplished healthcare providers in the world. Perhaps it would be a good subject for a book!

I started to read scientific papers on birth psychology. That's how I came across the ISPP and submitted a paper, "Tapping the Natal Memory Pool" to their next meeting. My paper was accepted, and I went to Salzburg, Austria, in March 1978 to present it at the 5th International Congress, International Study Group for Prenatal Psychology (ISPP). There I had the pleasure to meet Gustav Graber, Igor Caruso, Friedrich Kruse, Sep Schindler, and Peter Fodor Freybergh. It turned out that Peter and I were childhood friends and had lost touch many years ago. What a small world!

The same year, I presented a paper, "The Embryology of Consciousness" at APA and Societe Medico Psychologique, Paris, France, where I first met Michelle Odent.

After participating in the 6th International Congress of Obstetrics and Gynecology, West Berlin in Sep. 1980, my wife and I drove to Cagnes-sur-Mer in South of France and spent time with psychologist Ann Marie Saurel, director of The Tomatis Centre there. On another trip, we went to Holland and spent a lovely afternoon with Lietaert Peerbolte, author of *Psychic Energy.*

Based on all of these experiences and researching many scientific papers and books, I started to write the book that eventually was published as *The Secret Life of the Unborn Child*, (with John Kelly) in 1991.

Simon & Schuster, the publisher, sent me on a coast-to-coast book tour with the usual daily TV, radio, and newsprint interviews. In the course of my travels, I met many like-minded obstetricians, psychologists, midwives, and other healthcare professionals and academics. Most importantly, after a guest appearance on the Merv Griffin show in LA, I met Dr. David Chamberlain, and we started to correspond. David suggested we present a joint workshop on Birth Memories at the 1982 American Psychological Association Annual Meeting. Our proposal was quickly rejected. Disappointed, I rather impetuously said, "If they don't want us in their club, let's form our own."

By that time, I was corresponding with many scientists, obstetricians, psychologists, and others interested in early development. David also had a list of similarly inclined people which he shared with me. I called on these contacts when I organized the First International Congress on Pre- and Perinatal Psychology in 1983 in Toronto. This was before computers, and my secretary, God bless her, hand typed every letter of invitation and all subsequent correspondence.

About 500 people from all walks of life and from many countries attended the congress. It was a resounding success.

Immediately following the conclusion of the Congress, some of my colleagues and I had a meeting and founded the Pre- and Perinatal Psychology Association of North America (PPPANA), later renamed APPPAH. I was elected the Association's first president, and I continued in this role until 1991.

Two years later, under the chairmanship of David Chamberlain, we held our 2nd International Congress on pre-and perinatal psychology in San Diego, July 1985. We followed this by Congresses every two years in various locations in the USA.

In spring 1986, I met with executives of Human Sciences Press in New York and entered an agreement with them to publish our association's journal. The first issue of the *Pre- and Peri-Natal Psychology Journal* was published in fall 1986. I edited it from its inception until 1990. For the last ten years, I have acted as the journal's associate editor. The journal has been published quarterly since 1986.

In 1995, I initiated a program on pre- and perinatal psychology and health in the Department of Human Development at Saint Mary's University, Minneapolis, MN, and I met with great opposition from the conservative faculty of this program. Though we had many well-qualified students, the university shut down the program after three years.

However, the example and the curriculum inspired Dr. Martie Glenn to start the Santa Barbara Graduate Institute, at which I taught for eight years. The SBGI tried for many years and at great expense to become accredited as a university, but no matter how many hoops they jumped through, the authorities always came up with another one. Finally, Martie ran out of money and energy and closed down the facility. This event represented a huge loss to pre- and perinatal psychology.

In 1987 Human Sciences Press published the best papers given at the First PPP Congress in Toronto under the title *Pre- and Perinatal Psychology: An Introduction,* with me as the editor.

I followed this up with several books dealing with pre- and perinatal psychology, as follows:
Parenting Your Unborn Child, 1988 (also published in Japan).
Nurturing the Unborn Child (with Pamela Weintraub), United States and Canada, 1991 (Also published in Italy, Brazil, Japan, and Spain).

Tomorrow's Baby: The Art and Science of Parenting from Conception through Infancy, 2002 (Also published in Spain, Germany, Italy, Brazil, and Japan).

Pre-Parenting: Nurturing your Child from Conception, 2003 (The paperback edition of *Tomorrow's Baby*; also published in Japan).

I also contributed to three anthologies:
Verny, Thomas R. (2013). *Working with Pre- and Perinatal Material in Psychotherapy*, in **Die Pranatale Dimension in der Psychotherapie**, ed. Janus, Ludwig. Mattes Verlag, Heidelberg.

Verny, Thomas R. (2013). *The Pre & Perinatal Origins of Childhood and Adult Diseases and Personality Disorders* in **Lehrbuch der Prenatalen Psychologie**, ed. Evertz, Klaus; Janus, Ludwig and Linder, Rupert. Mattes Verlag, Heidelberg.

Verny, Thomas R. (2021). *The Inheritance of Change* in ***Change: Birthing & Parenting at Times of Crisis***. Eds. Olga Gouni, Jon RG Turner, Troya GN Turner.

Starting in 1981 with the publication of *The Secret Life of the Unborn Child*, like Johnny Appleseed, I set out to plant seeds of Prenatal and Perinatal Psychology throughout Canada, the

United States, Europe, South America, and Southeast Asia. I was also invited to present lectures and workshops in many countries.

My very worst experience at a conference occurred in Brussels at Koninklijke Belgische Vereniging Voor Gynecologie en Verloskunde, Affligem, Belgium, 1995, where I spoke on "Pre and Perinatal Obstetrical Procedures: A Psychosomatic Critique." I addressed what I called "gyne-gadgetry" like amniocentesis and fetal heart monitors. To say that it was not well received by the obstetricians present is an understatement. At least they rejected my message so very politely.

In 2004, in recognition of my contributions to the field of parenting and child rearing, *Mothering Magazine* named me one of their "living treasures." In 2005, the Santa Barbara Graduate Institute bestowed on me a Doctorate of Humane Letters (DHL). Recently, I have spoken at conferences in India, Italy, Spain, Chile, Brazil, and England.

When I wrote *The Secret Life of the Unborn Child*, almost forty years ago, I had a great deal of solid scientific evidence to back up the central premise of my book, namely that an unborn child is a sensing, feeling, conscious, and remembering being at least three months before birth. However, I had little or no scientific evidence to support cognition or memory of any kind reaching back further in time. Of course, given the rapidity of development and change in the biomedical sciences for the past decades, forty years is practically an aeon ago. Much of what is now known in cell biology, genetics, and, most importantly, epigenetics not only confirms my claims in *The Secret Life*, but also enables me to put forward the bold new concepts in my latest book, *The Embodied Mind*.

What set me on the path towards writing *The Embodied Mind* was an article I read seven years ago, reprinted from *Reuters*

Science News, entitled, "Tiny brain no obstacle to French civil servant."

The article outlines the store of a 44-year-old French man who, in July 2007, went to the hospital complaining of a mild weakness in his left leg. When doctors learned that the man had a spinal shunt removed when he was 14, they performed numerous scans of his head. What they discovered was a huge fluid-filled chamber occupying most of the space in his skull, leaving little more than a thin sheet of actual brain tissue. It was a case of hydrocephalus, or water in the brain. Dr. Lionel Feuillet of Hôpital de la Timone in Marseille was quoted as saying, "The images were most unusual... the brain was virtually absent." The patient was a married father of two children and worked as a civil servant apparently leading a normal life, despite having a cranium filled with spinal fluid and very little brain tissue.

To my surprise, I found in the medical literature an astonishing number of documented cases of adults who as children had parts of their brain removed to heal their persistent epilepsy. Following their hemispherectomies, most children showed not only an improvement in their intellectual capacity and sociability but also apparent retention of memory, personality, and sense of humor. Similarly, adults who have had hemispherectomies enjoyed excellent long-term seizure control and increased postoperative employability.

If people who lack a large part of their brain can function normally, or even relatively normally, then I believed there must exist some kind of a back-up system that can kick in when the primary system crashes. I devoted the next six years to the study of the medical and scientific literature, searching for clues to this puzzle.

While many scientists have contributed greatly to advancing science in their own areas of expertise, whether genetics or cellular biology, I have synthesized here these disparate findings, connected the dots, and in the process arrived at some significant new insights about the brain and the brain-mind relationship and how memory works.

The following is an extract of *The Embodied Mind*:
"It is imperative that we become aware of as many of our basic maladaptive urges and behaviors as possible and consciously try to overcome them. At the same time, it is imperative for our sake but especially for the benefit of our future children to live a good and healthy life. We shall vastly improve our lives and the lives of future generations by actively avoiding stress and anxiety as well as people who are critical or deceitful and instead befriend people who support and value us.

"We think, feel, and act with our body. We relate to the world with our body. Our mind is body bound. It is my hope that *The Embodied Mind* will help us gain more insights into who we are in relationship to ourselves, our loved ones, society, and the universe. It will motivate us to exercise our free will and encourage us to take responsibility for our own actions."

In April 2022, I will be starting a podcast, "Pushing Boundaries with Dr. Thomas R Verny, Pioneering Research, Breakthrough Discoveries, and Unconventional Ideas." It will feature dynamic interviews with established and emerging scientists, writers, and thinkers who work at the cutting edge of their disciplines. I view the world as a laboratory of ideas. I try to find the best, most intriguing of these and illuminate them with a bright and generous light. Stay tuned!

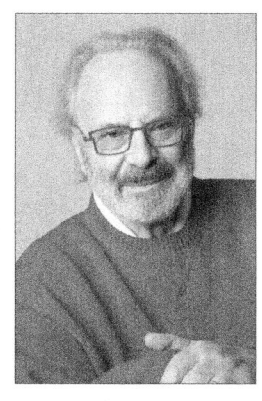

Thomas R. Verny, MD, DHL (Hon), DPsych, FRCPC, FAPA, is a Psychiatrist, author, and academic with a life-long interest in memory and the mind. Dr. Verny played a vital role in establishing globally the science of pre- and peri-natal psychology. He was the founding president of the Pre- and Peri-Natal Psychology Association of North America. Presently, he is Associate Editor of the Association's Journal. His book, *The Secret Life of the Unborn Child*, is available in 27 countries. Dr. Verny's most recent book, *The Embodied Mind,* focuses on cellular intelligence.

Website: https://www.trvernymd.com

The Embodied Mind (Oct. 5, 2021) Pegasus Press, New York, NY

On Amazon

On Amazon Canada

Chapter 3

DHYAN BABY AND GARBH SANSKAR

By Dr. N. Kalyani

My early dreams of becoming a doctor were shattered when my father suddenly died. I was only 11 years old. In the months of grief that followed, I missed my father greatly, but nothing could have prepared me for what was to come next. Now my dreams of dedicating my life to healing and serving seemed impossible. According to our customs, at the tender age of 13, I was to marry. The Indian tradition requires that widows who cannot provide an income for their family be confined to the home. I felt sad knowing that my mother would have to stay home for the rest of her life. She would never be allowed to leave the home, dress up, wear jewelry, or have a normal life. As for me, I married a man 18 years older than me who expected much the same of his wife.

My idea of marriage was naturally very naïve. I thought I would be free to go out, visit, and explore. This is something that other unmarried young girls were not allowed to enjoy. I had a lot to learn. The transition from childhood to married woman and then motherhood was cruelly abrupt. I now had a new family, a man I didn't know, and my in-laws to please. Neither of them took kindly to my ideas of studying and helping others. I felt alone, and being confined to my new home left me with little hope.

Married life was a challenge. By the time I was 15 years old, I had already had three abortions, including one without anesthetic. I was alone to face this excruciating physical and emotional suffering. But then at 16, I had my first baby. During my pregnancy I had the inspiration of doing something good for my baby. Now I was not alone. I hardly saw my husband, as he was busy and didn't take much care of me. My fertile imagination and passion now had its chance. I imagined I would unzip my stomach, take my baby out, play with him then put him back. I did this often and loved the interaction. I could feel that he responded to my love, care, and attention. I no longer felt alone.

It was during my first pregnancy that I took some secretarial and computer classes. Later, my son showed interest in technology and computer science. I understood that this was not by chance. My second baby, just two years later, was nine months old when she began to sing the mantras and chants that I often sang during my pregnancy. My daughter has become a beautiful musician and singer who is as passionate about helping others as I am.

My children are the masterpieces of my life. I had become so passionate about the connection between what happens during the time in the womb and later life. I began studying everything I could that would deepen my knowledge. I was lucky that Rajapalam, the town where I live in southern India, is a spiritual place. Many gurus and sages live here. I met many of them, and they encouraged me to learn about *garbh sanskar,* the ancient Vedic science on education in the womb.

During this intense learning phase, I went through some grueling experiences of endurance with some Buddhist saints in the nearby hills. They encouraged and prepared me to help others. They believed that we had to develop empathy to feel what others are feeling in order to really be of service to them. I learnt that it was not that easy to help human beings free themselves from suffering. I studied everything I could on the subjects of healing, energy, and human psychology and obtained my master's degree, followed by a doctorate in pregnancy therapy from the Indian Board of Cognitive Medicine. I am always eager to learn and develop myself.

When my children were 10 and 12 years old, my husband and I separated. This allowed me to continue working with the pregnant women I was now teaching. I soon came across women with severe trauma. Father Wilson, the Director of Anugraha Psychotherapy and Research Centre, helped me understand the deep emotional scars stemming from early childhood. "It's not so easy to help people to overcome this," he would say. I delved deeper into child psychology and became even more determined to understand how we can heal and, better still, prevent this suffering.

Doctors laughed at me when I went to talk to them in the Chennai and Coimbatore hospitals. The modern science of embryology provided some clues, but these were not sufficient to satisfy my driving passion and thirst for knowledge. The great Krishna Kumarji, founder of Ayurveda Pharmacy who had sacrificed his life to spread the Vedic sciences, took me under his wing. He introduced me to many sages from whom I continued to deepen my knowledge of this profound science. He opened my eyes to the necessity of teaching youth. It is during the time of puberty that the future generations are truly being formed. When girls start menstruating and boys begin producing sperm, they can begin this amazing preparation in mind, body, and spirit. This concept is so well explained in the Hindu sacred texts.

Our work with pregnant mothers and couples grew, and in 2002, the Dhyan Baby programme was born. *Dhyan* means "consciousness," so Dhyan Baby refers to a conscious baby. We also started teaching youth in the local schools, and my first book, *Successful Motherhood,* was published. Supporting mothers brings me so much joy. As childbirth educators, we also help mothers prepare for a natural, comfortable, and empowered birthing experience. We need to dehypnotize them from all the negative and frightening experiences they have heard or experienced. They need to learn how their body is perfectly designed to birth naturally. Giving birth is intended to be a joyful and loving celebration of life. However, it is all too often shrouded in fear and stress, which are often the causes of complications. There is so much to be done to educate not only mothers but also society on this subject.

The Dhyan Baby Foundation has conducted research over several years, and findings clearly show that there is a relationship between the care received by pregnant women (physical, psychological, and spiritual) and the child's intelligence, health, and wellbeing.

When babies are born, mothers also need support. We offer this support, which includes teaching them why and how to breastfeed their babies. Mother's milk is the perfect nourishment. A newborn baby's immune system is very immature; it needs to build up and adapt to the environment in which they live. If a baby is sick, the mother's milk provides the exact antibodies the baby needs to heal. No other milk or food can equal that which a mother can give her baby.

My family and I work together on our mission to serve mothers and their babies. My daughter is now also trained in Dhyan Baby and is also a childbirth educator, lactation consultant, and clinical music therapist. My son's business has started creating organic products for mothers and babies. It is so important that babies are not exposed to harmful chemicals which often go undetected and contribute to disease.

The continuation of care starting from preconception is essential. We started a preschool to provide this continuous care for our Dhyan babies. It is a place where our participating mothers can bring their children and connect with other children. Daily we witness the effects of a mother's pregnancy. Those who had a calm pregnancy have children who are calm and happy, whereas those who experienced difficult or stressful pregnancies have children who reflect this. Prevention is so much more effective than having to manage, heal, and correct things after.

We all know it is so important to build solid foundations for a building so that it lasts and doesn't collapse. There are architectural norms. But where are the norms for laying the foundations for the life of a human being who is going to live for perhaps a hundred years? The period of nine months in the mother's womb lays the foundation for physical, mental, and spiritual health. What the mother lives during this period is so crucial for the life-long health and blossoming of the child. It often determines whether the child can reach their full potential or not. The baby may not be in the mother's arms, but that doesn't mean she and the child can't already start getting to know each other and form a deep bond.

There is no other time in life where mother and baby are better able to communicate and share the most intimate feelings. A pregnant mother cannot hide her emotions from her unborn child. The womb is the first school for every man or woman. We will not lose much when a building collapses due to improper foundations. With additional investment, we can rebuild it.

But just imagine! After the birth of the baby, if we find that we have not given enough care during pregnancy to improve the baby's brain development, is it possible for you to ask the baby to return to the mother's womb to lay a new foundation? No!

The baby in utero is building its physical, emotional, mental, and spiritual bodies. They are learning about themselves, their parents, their environment, and about life. Let us help the baby to learn important things when in the mother's womb. These essential gifts last a lifetime. Programmes like Dhyan Baby offer scientifically, psychologically, and spiritually sound support for this.

During pregnancy, the mother spends every single second in a day with her baby. This is the only period during which her prenatal baby absorbs every single input, 100% without distraction. Now consider the analogy between a clay pot and shaping a baby in the womb. The shape of a clay pot can be determined only when the clay is wet. Once dried, the shape of the pot cannot be changed. If you try to change it, it will break.

Similarly, you can shape the IQ, EQ, SQ, and whatever you want of a baby when it is in the womb. After birth, it is similar to a dried pot. Characters can be shaped or fine-tuned by the expectant mother. The ten months the baby spends in the womb is the best period to educate a new human being about life.

The womb is not exactly the quietest place for the baby to hang out. The baby not only hears the sounds that the mother makes – including her stomach growling, hiccups, or burps – but also the outside sounds like music and cars. Babies react to sounds by kicking or shifting around. Around the seventh month, the developing baby's heart rate slows down slightly whenever his mother is speaking. This indicates that the mother's voice has a calming effect. Newborn babies can recognize their mother and father's voices. Until the seventh month, the baby's eyes are closed. Then prenatal babies are able to see. However, they see only darkness inside the womb. Whenever the mother is outside and allows bright light to fall on her belly, the baby sees it and reacts to avoid the effects of the bright light. Studies using ultrasound prove that they gradually open and close their eyes more and more as they come closer to being born.

The quality of food eaten by the mother is so important. The baby also tastes the food that the mother has eaten. There is evidence to show they distinguish between bitter, sweet, or sour flavors in the amniotic fluid. Ultrasound studies have shown babies licking the placenta and uterine wall. "The more varied a mother's diet during pregnancy and breastfeeding, the more likely that the infant will accept a new food," says Julie Mennella, Ph.D., a biopsychologist at the Monell Chemical Senses Center, in Philadelphia.

Babies develop their sense of smell in utero. After birth, they use smell rather than vision to identify their mother. All this goes to show that a baby isn't just passively waiting to be born. He's already building important skills and developing a bond with the most important person in his life – his mother. The fast-developing neurons of the brain learn to absorb any information that comes its way. Science now reveals that this is the best period for giving any kind of input and shaping the future of the baby.

The unutilized brain cells are wasted. It is up to the expectant mother to decide whether to utilize the baby's cells fully or to waste them. Mothers have the possibility to use this time consciously by giving positive input to her developing baby. Every mother should know how and be supported to make use of this time to give a magnificent human being to society and the world.

My dream is actually becoming a reality. I have become a doctor, one who truly participates in the prevention of disease. We hope this awareness will grow and that mothers and their babies will take a central place in society as it was in the time of the Vedas. When we look after mothers and their babies, children will grow up healthy, happy, intelligent, and enlightened. Together with the Birthing The New Humanity movement, we are helping to create a conscious humanity that starts with the beginning of life. This is the only sure way of assuring that our global family will blossom and that every child will be able to reach their full potential and thrive.

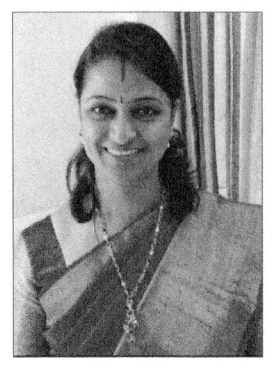

Dr. N. Kalyani founded Dhyan Baby prenatal education in 2000. Her programme is based on the concept that every child is a blessed child. She helps couples to have a conscious conception, healthy pregnancy, a happy birth, and the best motherhood experience possible. She has impacted some 200,000 school and college students and has touched the lives of 20,000 couples. She is an advisory council member of BTNH.

Chapter 4

PRENATAL MEMORY:
Global Peace Starts with a Peaceful Family Environment

By Dr. Akira Ikegawa
Edited and Translated by Yuko Igarashi

I first learned about Prenatal Memory from a book titled, "Creating the Value of Life" by Fumihiko Iida, which describes regression hypnosis. I first encountered the idea that the baby in the womb has consciousness in this book. All OB/GYN doctors had been taught that babies are unconscious and blind at birth, so at that time, I didn't believe in the idea that babies could see or understand while in the womb. I normally would have disregarded the topic, but as I was an obstetrician and I was curious about the contents, I finished the book very quickly. The book offered many examples and references, and so I started reading all the references I could get my hands on. I then experienced a drastic reduction in birth problems and even postpartum parenting issues when I implemented birth with the assumption that the baby has consciousness. For this reason, I am convinced that, if we obstetricians and midwives who are involved in childbirth can change the way we think about childbirth, we can achieve a different kind of childbirth and parenting.

When asking the staff at my clinic if they knew about the consciousness of an unborn baby, two of them responded that they knew about it. One staff member testified that her grandson recalled experiences from the womb, and the other said that her nephew had memories. I decided to conduct a full-scale investigation. First, I conducted a questionnaire survey of pregnant women who visited my clinic, a nearby midwifery clinic, and some kindergartens. I collected 79 questionnaires, and the results were announced in 2001 in the Japanese Medical and Dental Practitioners for the Improvement of Medical Care.

In 2002, Suwa City hosted a lecture called "Childcare University" as part of a 50-year post-war commemorative project to revitalize the town. The project gathered professionals involved in childcare, and Ikegawa was invited as a lecturer. After the event, when I told the head of the kindergarten that he wanted to conduct a questionnaire survey at the largest kindergartens in Suwa city, and the head of the kindergarten told me, "We cannot make decisions at our level. Please contact Suwa city council for permission." Then I contacted the city official to conduct the survey at a kindergarten from the city, and I was able to obtain the city's cooperation and conducted the survey among all childcare facilities in Suwa. I distributed 1,773 questionnaires consisting of 85 questions to all the childcare facilities in Suwa and received 838 (45%) responses, which were then analyzed for statistical purposes.

Introducing Prenatal Memory to the World
The results from Suwa City were presented at a conference of The International Federation of Gynecology and Obstetrics (Federation Internationale de Gynecologie et de Obstetrique - FIGO) in Chile in 2003.

That same year, I conducted a questionnaire survey of 1,828 guardians in Shiojiri City in August 2003 and collected 782 (42.8%) and compiled the data.

While researching papers on Prenatal Memory, I found a Japanese person who was a member of The Association for Prenatal and Perinatal Psychology and Health (APPPAH) and contacted her to request a copy of the articles. I sent the results of the survey in 2003 to a clinical psychologist named Hideko Sato, who immediately introduced me to Dr. Chamberlain, and I joined APPPAH. I presented my article with data compiled from the cities of Shiojiri and Suwa to the APPPAH in 2005. The following data is an excerpt from a paper published in JOPPPAH (ISSN1097-8003), 20(2), winter 2005,121-133.

My research revealed that Prenatal Memory has been most often shared by children between the ages of 2 to 4 (**2<3- 142, 3<4- 187**), and it dramatically drops after 4 (4<5- 56, 5<6- 23, 6<7- 5). The number of children who show Prenatal Memory gradually decreases, and the retention rate drops drastically from 40% (4 years old) to 20% (6 years old).

I personally interviewed Dr. Chamberlain at the APPPAH's International Congress in 2006, and it was a great opportunity for me to learn that other countries are also working in the same field.

From Prenatal Memory to Education of the Heart
Originally, I was not very interested in spirituality. I believed in animistic beliefs, blessings, and superstitions in folk tales. I have always had a sense of awe of the natural world and a sense of indigenous beliefs.

I had never talked about the spiritual world or the soul, but I became interested in these topics through my exploration of children's education. In general, obstetricians and gynecologists have a goal of making births safe and reducing the mortality rate, so they have not focused on how children should be educated. However, the small Japanese midwifery clinics, just like general practitioners in town, allow us to keep an eye on the growth process of the first child throughout the process of the second and third children's birth. For this reason, some of my patients have been coming to my clinic for as long as ten years. Based on my interactions with these patients over the years, I became very interested in how the babies born in my clinic would grow up. When I learned about the concept of Prenatal Memory and decided to adopt this concept, I was astonished to learn what the children were describing.

The following is an essay written by the staff member's grandson, and this is the first encounter of Prenatal Memory in my life. The essay was written by a first-grade boy:

- A kitchen knife came through my mom's stomach.
- A man with white clothes was wearing glasses and he grabbed my foot and took me out from a bag.
- I was crying because the rubber tube came through my nose, and I was choking.
- When I told my mother, she said it was a dream, but I thought it was real, not a dream.

Normally, when a c-section is performed, the baby comes out head first, but in this essay, it is written that the baby was "grabbed by the legs". An obstetrician would have known that the child was born breech the moment he/she read this, but even the mother did not know the fact that breech babies are born feet first during a c-section. How does a first grader know a fact that even his mother would not know?

When he wrote that the suction through the rubber tube in the nostril was choking, I felt that it was something that a person would not normally know if they didn't experience it. The doctor uses amniotic fluid suction so that the baby does not suffer, and the fact that he felt relieved to be able to breathe after the suction is in agreement with the doctor's view, but the fact that the child wrote that the procedure felt choking made me ponder that perhaps he vividly remembers what he experienced.

Later on, I became interested in talking to a baby properly, so I asked a renowned dowser for instructions. I asked about their date of birth, and about 70-80% of the time the answers were correct. I began to have a strong sense that the baby is indeed conscious, but it was difficult to communicate this fact to the parents who visited my clinic.

The Secret to Effectively Communicating the Prenatal Memory

Even though I had tried explaining to people that, babies are in fact conscious and that they can remember things in the womb, they didn't accept it very easily. I thought about how I could effectively communicate Prenatal Memory, and I decided that it was important to help the parents recognize that the baby is conscious first. The first thing I did was ask parents to talk to their babies in utero, but they said they were too embarrassed to communicate. However, I thought it was really important to encourage parents to talk to their babies, so I started by assertively saying, "The baby knows!" and emphasizing the fact that they are conscious beings. When the father talked to the baby, the mothers' moods were especially soothed, which I think was due to the difference in the feelings of the couples and the fact that many couples did not communicate with each other. Japanese wives were very considerate and withheld their emotions from their husbands.

I explained, "If a baby is born to a father who talked to the baby in the womb, the baby will smile at their father after birth. If the father doesn't talk to the baby in the womb, then the baby will cry when the father holds the baby after birth. Do you want your baby to smile or cry?" Gradually, maternity blues were decreased significantly.

In other words, when you tell the parents about Prenatal Memory, the parents will be able to sense that the baby is in fact conscious. Through this process, couples, parents, and children can communicate and understand each other's feelings, and the family bond is strengthened.

I feel that prenatal education, as it is commonly called, is a one-sided provision of information given to children from the perspective of adults. I propose that, by utilizing Prenatal Memory, we will be able to enhance the circulation of information between the parent and the child through imagery, and the bond between the family will become stronger as it grows. By engaging in a pleasurable dialog as a couple from the time of pregnancy, we can also practice two-way communication with the baby.

Will Family Relationships Change if Prenatal Memory Becomes Known Globally?

By understanding Prenatal Memory, we can realize that we are not just physical beings, but multidimensional beings with minds and souls.

If we have relationships based on Prenatal Memory, heart-to-heart communication will occur. Consequently, you will be able to accept diversity and acknowledge the differences between you and the other, which will prevent conflict. If the couple is having an argument, it means that the couple is experiencing a conflict of opinion. In other words, the next generation needs to be able to solve problems by respecting themselves while also respecting the other person, and I believe that the education of the next generation will nurture this idea between parents and their children from the prenatal period when the baby is still in the womb.

I have come to discover through my research on Prenatal Memory that children can only speak at the knowledge level of their parents and that the level of knowledge of adults is limited. In other words, if parents heighten their level of knowledge and information, the details of the children's Prenatal Memory will amplify and evolve to match the new and improved level of the parents.

We tend to perceive that empathizing with others is a good thing, but we often suppress our own feelings in order to please others. Are we expressing our thoughts without being too emotional? It is important to acknowledge what the other person may be thinking and try to overcome problems one by one while also respecting diversity in the process.

I believe that communicating such diversity from the time of conception will surely change the outcome of childbirth.

Let's Move Forward with Our Global Initiative, Birthing The New Humanity!

The world will be a more peaceful, mutually accepting, and diverse place if we could change the way we interact with the 1.6 billion unborn babies and newborns. These children are 20% of the world's population, estimated to be 8 billion by 2024. There are about 6,900 languages spoken in the world, and there are 1.6 billion people who speak Chinese, English, and Spanish alone. I believe it is possible to reach 20 percent of the world's population through these languages. If the concept of Prenatal Memory is accepted, I believe that we can build a peaceful world. I will continue to do my best to achieve the goal of building a peaceful society together with citizens of the world who embrace the thriving human family and planet. Will you join us by supporting us through our global initiative, Birthing The New Humanity?

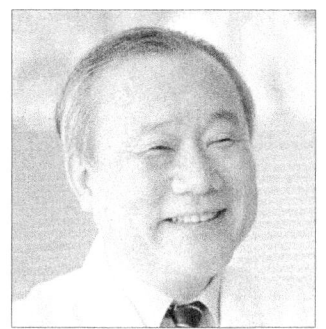

Akira Ikegawa, Director of the Ikegawa Clinic, is a respected healthcare professional and author of more than 80 books. With an extensive background in the research of Prenatal Memory, he delivers lectures globally about his research on holistic childbirth and conscious parenting to create a harmonious lifestyle for the thriving human family and planet.

Yuko Igarashi International Coordinator – Prenatal Memory Education Association Japan is currently working to help create a sustainable future by spreading the concept of Prenatal Memory. https://akira-ikegawa.com/en/

Chapter 5

IT'S THE BABY'S BIRTH

By Janel Mirendah

You were the baby at your birth. That seems like such an obvious statement, but I want you to really think about that for the moment. When you were born it was your experience of coming from the spirit world to the human world. It was your birth. Pause, take a deep breath. Come back to this breath anytime you feel sensation or triggered as I tell you my story of coming to this world and why I live for the moment when a person realizes on a deep, visceral level, that "Oooh myyy God, that was ME! I was the baby. I have my story to tell."

When a person truly gets that they were the baby, they can no longer do harm to babies doing what is seen now as normal, routine care in obstetrics. Everything I do as a craniosacral therapist, filmmaker, and artist is focused on supporting people to access their early baby self and to integrate their birth trauma. This is how we create a peaceful life, family, and world.

In the opening scene of the 1991 movie, *City Slickers*, Mitch Robbins, played by Billy Crystal, is awakened at 5:15 am by a phone call from his mother. He is still groggy. She gleefully says, "It's September 8, 1952. We are driving back from your Aunt Marcia's. My water breaks. Your father jumps the divider ..." By now Mitch is mouthing the words to his mother's story ... "of the Saw Mill River Parkway and races me to the doctor's hospital." She is laughing, and Mitch is comically imitating her. "And at 5:16, out you came!" She laughs and sighs, "Happy birthday, darling. Here's your father," who says something about a physical ailment and then, "Here's your mother."

I love that scene. It reminds me of my mom and dad, except my dad also has his story about my birth because he was there in the room and witnessed my arrival. He was not excluded like 96% of fathers in 1956, left to sit in the waiting room or at the bar. Today, men still have a story of being disempowered but now they witness the obstetric abuse, and unfortunately, they still have no support to process their experiences. In modern society, we are expected to accept traumatizing medicalized birth as normal and to accept that "the baby is fine."

Babies are not fine. Watching their fathers being disempowered at birth led me to create a film, *The Other Side of the Glass: a birth film for and about men*, released in June of 2013. The man's experience of becoming a father was mostly ignored prior to my fundraising trailer that went viral within a day of release in the fall of 2009. It started a much-needed conversation about a man's experience at his baby's birth and his need for validation that he is having his own experience. He is witnessing his partner and baby's traumatic experience.

Men across the US shared with me their experiences of witnessing the births of their babies. They said it was "like being in a war zone," that they were powerless on "the other side of the glass," even when they were present at hospital births and expected to participate and protect. The film challenges viewers to see that the father is unable to protect his partner and baby while he is experiencing his baby's birth.

About *The Other Side of the Glass*, Pragya Upadhyay, Child Psychologist said, "It starts out bringing forth the perspectives and feelings of men about the birth and how birth impacts them as a person. How it impacts their own self-esteem and personal relationships, then it goes further by revealing the larger impact of this medically created helplessness. This does not only affect the man as an individual but also extends to the family, community, nations, and the entire world. The film also shows how our current world of disharmony, imbalance and violence is just a reflection of the inner state of violated and traumatized humanity!"

Through the stories of fathers, midwives, doulas, and doctors, the overall theme of the film is that the foundation established by the mother-baby connection at birth is neurologically critical for creating a humanity that is in thriving (love) mode, rather than in survival (fear) mode. The neural understanding of the mother-baby development and connection is introduced. The film focuses on the needs of newborns at birth and the impact on the family and society for not understanding this and making no effort to meet those needs.

The film implores caregivers (doctors, nurses, and midwives) to be the ones to protect the mother-baby dyad and father in the hospital and home setting, and to protect skin-to-skin at birth. Stop harming babies. The outcome I want from my film is for people to become aware of the critical need to see birth as a vital experience and to protect birth for all humans. The film supports men to realize that they cannot protect their child and partner at birth in the modern patriarchal-based maternity system, but men can engage outside of their birth experience to protect all women and babies by addressing their local hospitals and their county and state policymakers.

I implore men to join together with others in their community and educate themselves with scientific data about what human babies need and about the physiologic, mammalian birth that women are built to experience. I want them to organize in groups and go to their local hospitals to meet with administrators and obstetricians to demand that their hospital practice evidence-based physiological birth with a priority of keeping the mother-baby dyad together.

People often ask me what inspired me to make a film about fathers. First, my father was present at my birth in 1956 when only 4% of men were even "allowed" in birthing rooms. My dad was also present at all of my five siblings' births from 1949-1970. Second, in my study of birth trauma healing I realized I had my own story as the baby. Did you notice in the story of Mitch's birth told by his mother that she said, "*my* water broke," "your father races *me*" to the hospital, and "then you came out"? The membranes, the placenta, and the cord are all the baby's, not the mother's. Even the amniotic fluid is produced mainly by the baby. It's the baby's body and the baby's birth from the mother. Humanity must get this change of perspective. It's the baby's birth, the mother's experience of giving birth, and the father or others' experience of witnessing the birth.

My birth was my birth, and it defined me for life in myriad ways. In the womb and at birth, I was a sentient and aware being. I was learning my mother's language and her voice, my father's, and my siblings'. At birth, my brain had billions of neurons already firing and wiring up everything I saw, felt, heard, smelled, and tasted. It is today all stored in my preverbal emotional brain, in my amygdala in my limbic system, as implicit, sensory, and emotional body memory. In trauma-informed therapy practices, we now know how to access this so the adult self can hear their own baby story and put language to their experience.

Our early brain functions much like computers do in ones and zeros, firing or not firing. The limbic system becomes the emotional "operating system" that runs the programs that are installed during childhood. It is in critical development starting in the last trimester and continuing through around age two. The limbic brain is the emotional and sensory brain. At birth, the human baby is 150 times more sensitive than at any other time. This is nature's design to create attachment between the mother and baby.

I knew in my body and my preverbal brain that my own birth was traumatic and that my dad had been powerless to protect me and my mom. I knew deeply that my birth defined me and that it defined my dad as a young man and as a husband, father, and human being. My birth was very traumatic and like most babies I was never able to tell my story, to be heard, felt, and held in this deep emotional wound. I never heard my dad talk about his feelings until I interviewed him for the film.

Through interviewing my dad and fathers around the United States, I began to understand that fathers shouldn't be expected to protect their loved ones in the hospital or during home births. Fathers need to experience love, joy, and connection during the birth, to feel the love hormone oxytocin flow, not be overwhelmed with fear, anger, panic, guilt, and shame. Fathers should not be in the flight-fight-freeze state when welcoming their baby.

Prior to the film, I did the two-year Castellino Prenatal and Birth Therapy program experiencing the process that works within the limbic system. During my healing experience, I learned that I was struggling to live. I have a very strong constitution for living. My experience coming to this planet was painful and I dissociated. I left my body to get through it. I became a survivor. I was too wounded to cry and my mother experienced me as "a good baby." Via the training, I grieved, embraced, and integrated my own story as a baby.

A gift from my traumatic birth, the near-death experience, and never fully embodying was the ability to dance between the worlds. I was clairsentient and clairaudient as a child. I was fortunate that my mother did what we know now as attachment mothering; I was breastfed, carried, and placed to sleep by her in the bed. I was her third child, and my mom was happy she was able to quit her work and stay home with me. However challenging my dissociation and sensitivity was for me, it was also mediated by my mother's attachment mothering.

Attachment mothering was the focus of the research of Dr. Harry Harlow in the '50s, and I was blessed to meet him in 1974, a year before I had my first child at 18.5. He validated my mother's mothering, and I was determined to do the same. My son's birth was also very traumatic, but even so, the moment I had him in my arms, I experienced an other-worldly spiritual moment in the chaos.

I was in awe that this beautiful creature whose eyes held the universe came out of me! He was mine, but he wasn't. He was another person. Another soul. Although separate from me, he was still me. I knew deeply that I brought him into this world, but I did not own him. This amazingly beautiful soul was entrusted to me. I loved and wanted him from the very first moment I knew of him. Gazing into his eyes at birth, I stepped into the responsibility of mothering. Like with my mother, my son and I experienced a strong maternal connection through breastfeeding.

My experience of my son's birth began my internal inquiry about how birth surely defines us. Meanwhile, I worked in multiple systems attempting to support mothers and children and to end child abuse. By 1998, I had worked my way to the top level in New York state when I was directing a program to address the vagaries of the failing mother-child systems of support. It was my dream job to stop systemic abuse and change the system from the inside! In reality, it turned out to be a nightmare, because the system did not want to change. Systems are abusive and self-perpetuating. I left as a whistleblower, and I spent two months in a painful, dark night of the soul.

After two months, I attended an infant massage training. The trainer focused on birth trauma, and there I was introduced to the work of David Chamberlain, Bruce Lipton, and William Emerson, thought leaders in birth psychology and soul consciousness. The trainer had us think about a personal challenge. Panic and procrastination came to me. The next day in class, while processing this, I experienced a visceral-level understanding that my cord trauma was related to my feelings. The baby moves forward and faces lack and death, pulls back, and feels failure. Emerson calls this "completion ambivalence."

At that moment, I heard the Hallelujah chorus. Seriously. The clouds parted and the sun came out when I realized that I am the baby who experienced the cord wrapped around my neck 2.5 times and the forceps that forcefully pulled me out. Now I knew I could heal. Shortly after I started craniosacral therapy training. I realized immediately that obstetrics IS the first system of abuse. Since then, I have sought to end the abuse of the obstetric system and to help those who are harmed to heal. This is my life's mission, supporting people to realize that they were the baby and to access and integrate their own story.

Through my craniosacral work, I became conscious of my life-long gift of clairsentience and clairaudience that I had shut down. It came back to me while communicating with babies. The first baby whose voice I heard told me he was unable to move from breech position because he would compromise the cord. When doctors attempted a version (manually moving a baby), he fiercely resisted. He was born by cesarean. I saw the baby from my car a few weeks later, asleep on his father's chest and I didn't see him again until he was two and a half.

I was at a meeting when I heard the mom call out my name. They were at the other end of a long hallway. The boy stopped suddenly, looked, and then ran to me. He jumped on my feet, and facing me, his feet climbed up my body and he did a full backward flip. He was showing me what he had needed to do to turn. I said, "Ooooh. It was like that. I see." Later he sang my name in the car all the way home so his mother booked another session. We worked on his "oppositional behavior" related to the medical attempt to turn him. He told *his* story, and his mother listened with *her* ears, heart, and full body. This experience shifted their relationship. My experience with this baby is one of the many relationships in which these souls have led me to my therapeutic process to help individuals process their birth stories.

It is challenging and scary to hear our baby's experience of birth. I have developed a process I call Soul Portraits to support people to begin gently and safely to explore their origin experience of conception, embryonic stages of life, labor, birth, and early infancy. I can help you process your origin and birth story and how it impacts your life today. I channel your story of pain, loss, and separation into a beautiful image of joy, bliss, and connection that you can color or meditate upon. It works in the limbic system so you can process your story gently and safely in order to live the happy peaceful life we all crave.

You can find *The Other Side of the Glass* and my current artwork at www.JanelMirendah.com.

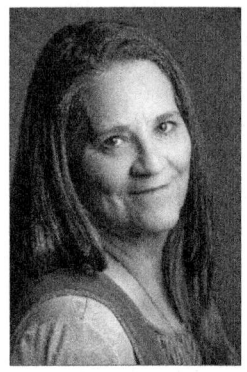

Janel Mirendah is a filmmaker, a spiritual guide, a therapist, a researcher, an activist, a mother, and an artist. Weaving all of these gifts together, she is a Babykeeper, one who keeps the soul's journey of coming into human form through a woman and a man as the focus of birth. She believes we can create the world we seek if we stop harming humans at birth and help those who have been harmed – most of us – to heal their early baby self and integrate their birth trauma. This is how we create a peaceful life, family, and world.

Chapter 6

HEALING PRENATAL TRAUMA

By Dr. Francois Gerland (*hc*)

"Dad! Is it really you…?"

"Yes, son, I'm here. Get ready. I'm taking you on a trip." My father stands at the main door of our French Pyrenees house. He smiles, looking confident that I will follow him without hesitation.

To my surprise, I hear myself asking, "What type of car do you have?"

"A Golf."

"OK, that will do!" I say, obviously ready to leave everything behind, including my beloved wife, without a clue about what my father has in mind.

"Does this mean you're not mad at me anymore?" he asks.

Once again, my answer seems to come from some unknown part of my consciousness: "Oh no, not anymore. Everything's fine now because you came back!"

My heart is about to explode with joy, and it probably would if not for my nagging concern about leaving everything behind for an unknown destination.

We get into the car, and just as we begin to drive off, I wake up with vivid memories of this scene that seemed more real than life. He had been here, and he asked me to follow him, which felt like the most obvious thing to do. But it was a dream. No Volkswagen Golf was parked in front of the house. The man whose arms I so wished would embrace me was nowhere to be seen.

Why did he ask if I was mad at him? Never had I consciously been angry at him for having left me behind.

November 21, 1964
My dad, 40 years old and solid as a rock, played ping-pong with a priest. My dad's doctor had expressed concern about his two daily packs of cigarettes and heavy consumption of strong black coffee, but my 11-year-old self didn't know anything about that. I was busy admiring my hero, skillfully reaching for a very tricky shot under the corner of the table. But instead of coming back to the game, he kept falling further and further, until he lay flat on the ground, expressionless, under the table. Later that day, my mother simply told me that I no longer had a father.

Why on earth would I be angry with him? After all, he didn't do anything wrong, and I can't imagine he died on purpose. But what I didn't realize and would only learn years later is that the human being has a subconscious mind. When a child loses his source of security, strength, and loving guidance, lots of things happen in the hidden depth of his being.

Ever since I gained the ability to express myself, I talked about airplanes. At age 11, I already so wanted to be a pilot that my teacher had called my mother to tell her that my vocation was basically set in stone. But how would I ever become a pilot without a dad to guide me?

To ease the deep void in my heart, I decided to turn to my other Father, the one who can do anything, even though I was told that He lives "up there," and His existence is loaded with dogma and very strange ways of treating humanity. Living close to a Franciscan convent, I also had developed a deep admiration for St. Francis of Assisi. The decision was made. I would become a priest... a Franciscan, of course!

But what about flying?

The answer was obvious: I would be a priest-pilot! Flying in a robe shouldn't be that difficult, after all.

As you might expect, this aero-mystical fantasy wouldn't last long. One day, some clumsy words declared in a catechism class led me to abandon my commitment to God, religion, priesthood, and even faith. Aviation would be my way, my god, my source of joy. Girls were interesting, too, but totally unreachable for a fatherless boy with self-esteem issues.

The same void in my heart never went away, but I certainly didn't have the time or means to fill it. I was working hard to achieve my dream.

Five years later, on a beautiful morning, I gazed at a small tree in a semi-dreamy state. Little did I know that this simple moment and 5 short words would give instant meaning to my life:

"But, of course God exists."

Did the voice come from my head, my heart, my soul? Had the tree just talked to me? The message was as clear as crystal, completely soft and yet as powerful as truth itself. Nothing would ever be the same after these few seconds of bliss.

I knew that this God wasn't the one my instructors had tried to teach me. A new consciousness had opened – I wouldn't be a priest-pilot but a spiritualist-pilot! Of course, I had many problems to solve and many questions to answer. What was this strange anguish I felt? Why was I so afraid of public opinion? Why was I so attracted to some people and repulsed by others? Why did I feel on top of the world after some meditation, only to crash down later with everyday thoughts, feelings, and actions?

Was I the only one with these questions? Everybody else seemed so sure of themselves. Why did I have all of these doubts and uncertainties? Only after meeting my spiritual teacher, Master Omraam Mikhaël Aïvanhov, did I realize the validity of this questioning. He gave the most precise answers to all of them, including ones I had never asked. Finally, life started to make sense. The God he presented to me was the source of all perfection, the only Real Existence, not only around me but also within me. Another huge door had opened; the work could start. I knew that the void would be replaced by plenitude and my fears replaced by unconditional love. Wisdom would enlighten the darkest parts of my soul. My interest for the subconscious and superconscious mind grew fast and would never leave me.

These wonderful Teachings made complete sense to me. The deep work really started, however, when my spiritual partner, who later became my beautiful wife, appeared in my life. Through the miracle of love and polarity, we discovered that the most hidden parts of our subconscious mind are as obvious to the other as the nose on our face. Discovering the wonders of each other's soul was a display of outstanding beauty that brought us a deep understanding of what alchemists call the "magic mirror." At first, the experience felt like drinking the elixir of immortal life, and it certainly gave us a taste of what it means to be "on top of the mountain."

But magic mirrors aren't just meant to show beauty; they actually show the truth. One after the other, my deepest wounds were exposed in full light, and the pain I felt upon refusing to see them was at times overwhelming. Trained in a modern western society, I was accustomed to seeking pleasure and running away from pain, not knowing that the latter held the key to finding who we truly are: an eternal consciousness that will never be affected by the ups and downs of superficial life. It expands through every experience.

Today, as I look back on some of the most difficult times we have lived, I understand the concept of the "wounded healer." I couldn't accompany my clients through their deepest trauma if I hadn't experienced these areas of consciousness, through which we all feel misunderstood, inadequate, unworthy, abandoned, lonely, and only able to see the future as a big, long, grey tunnel.

"It is in great sorrow that sublime love is born," said the great Bulgarian Master Peter Deunov. When I read this sentence for the first time, I felt shock and sincerely hoped there was another way to find such love. What I hadn't understood is that there was actually another way to **suffer**. A conscious suffering enables us, instead of fleeing our sorrows, to look at them directly, and then they start opening like blossoming roses. The secret of this opening is to devote our fearless attention to what's really happening inside of us without falling into the trap of trying to change outside circumstances and people in order to feel better.

As I work with the subconscious mind in daily practice, my buried memories start reaching my consciousness, and it feels natural to experience the early origin of my dysfunctional state. I had never dared to accept the possibility that I could have been angry at my father, until I connected with the 11-year-old boy inside me who had been "abandoned" by the one he loved so much. Yes, I had been angry, and yes, it was okay to be angry. I surrounded that boy with unconditional love and made him aware that my father could be with me as often as I invited him into my consciousness and heart.

I then discovered that this abandoned feeling had started long before 1964, actually even before I was born. When my young mother found herself pregnant much before the wedding day, it meant absolute catastrophe for her devoted Catholic parents. She had committed a terrible sin, to the shame of the whole family, not to mention that this brilliant student would never earn her college degree. The baby inside her received her despair, sadness, and even deep anger against the situation as well as her parents' rigid attitude. I was not wanted. I came at the wrong time, I didn't belong, I shouldn't have been here. Logically, the birth happened just a few months after the wedding in May 1953. My birth would only be announced to the extended family in August. In the meantime, the fruit of the shameful act had to "disappear" far away from Paris. The most important moments of my life were devoid of the joy and bliss that many other children experience at such times.

The discovery of how I felt during the first 12 months of my existence, from the moment of conception, came to me as an electroshock, which opened the doors to working on my prenatal trauma and helping many people, including future parents, to heal theirs.

As you may have learned in other chapters of this book, the prenatal period is of fundamental significance to every human being. How parents, and especially mothers, live during these sacred nine months will create the basis of their child's intelligence, emotional stability, health, and wellbeing. Happy parents create luminous children. This is why it is so important to have cleared as much trauma as possible before conceiving a child.

So how does this work? How can we handle the traumas we aren't even conscious of?

The first step is to de-dramatize them. The optimistic ending of many fairy tales, "and they lived happily ever after," is excellent wishful thinking, but it doesn't reflect the actual lives of most people. A perfect life isn't one in which nothing wrong ever happens. Problems are here to help us grow, and trauma can be seen as a problem that occurred too early. However, it's never too late to address them!

Once you have understood that Unconditional Love is stronger than anything else in the universe, you can bring this love into where it is most needed: in the parts of the inner world you've avoided all your life while feeling unable to face them.

Letting your body relax and breathing deeply, you can contact the child inside you who carries a burden far too heavy for him or her to shoulder. This child needs five very basic things: safety, trust, understanding, love, and guidance. If you can give these few things to a physical child, you can surely give them to your inner child.

I was stunned to learn that children who had been victims of severe abuse were often far more hurt by the betrayal or absence of support from their parents than by the abuse itself. You can fix this by being present for your inner child and possibly becoming their champion. Your wonderful imagination will help you contact this child and feel the warm embrace between you. It's even possible to imagine yourself becoming this child for just a moment and receiving the support and unconditional love from the caring adult holding the younger you in their arms.

Revisiting my story – what did I do for my inner unborn child? I advanced toward him as if I was approaching the most precious object in the world. I told him that he had been conceived at the perfect moment and that I wouldn't let anyone criticize him or his very existence. I assured him that, as of now, I would be with him whenever he needed me.

When I start feeling misunderstood, unworthy, criticized, or abandoned, I know that my inner little boy needs me. I'll then sit with him for a while, letting him know that I am here for him. Soon, a gentle feeling of warmth and safety fills up my heart, and I can deal with the triggering situation without adding additional stress.

It takes very little time to experience some deep relief in areas in which suffering has reigned for years. Nevertheless, please be aware that you will always have more to do and learn. The widening of consciousness is infinite work through which we must practice enjoying the ride, not just the goal. The destiny of humanity is immense, and it is a waste to believe we have already reached perfection.

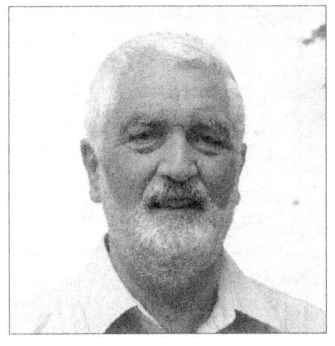

Dr. Francois Gerland (*hc*) is the co-founder of Birthing The New Humanity and BirthTheChange®. He was born in Paris in 1953 and is passionate about understanding our human and divine natures. A brilliant hypnotherapist and trainer, Dr. Gerland has combined his career as an airline pilot with his work as an international speaker and advocate for prenatal life at the United Nations. He was awarded an honorary doctorate in holistic medicine.

Chapter 7

HOW BIRTH AFFECTS LIFE

By Alex Florschutz, MA

Every human being starts life inside a woman's body, and we enter the world (in most cases) through her genitals. However, a woman is often controlled, violated, and disempowered during birth due to the reliance on a medical system that acts like a supreme being to be obeyed, for fear of putting oneself and one's baby at risk.

My question is this: How can pregnancy and birth as a deeply instinctual experience and part of nature, spanning millions of years, and an art form with which we are rapidly losing touch, be trusted once again? How do we reconnect back to the ancient natural life cycles of the human being and translate them, in a positive way, to our time? I believe birth is a feminist issue!

Women have the power to reclaim birth and what is done to their bodies. Through my journey, I discovered that a new positive birth paradigm is desperately needed, and art can be a powerful antidote.

* * *

In 1998, I was living in the beautiful island of Bali, Indonesia, where – in a nutshell – I met a handsome Balinese man, got married, and conceived my son. I loved Bali, because it gave me the clear message that pregnancy, birth, motherhood, and the feminine were revered, and women are fully supported by family and culture. The Balinese live much more in the flow and try to live meaningful, balanced lives. They sincerely believe that human beings come from the spiritual world and, when they die, they return to their ancestors to prepare to be reborn once again. It's the cycle of life, death, and rebirth.

However, when I was 6 months pregnant, my husband and I moved back to the UK, where I gave birth. Here I was met with a very different picture: fear, danger, and a medical procedure for every eventuality.

We are very lucky to have great medical care here in the UK when it is needed, because a live baby and mother are paramount, but I never learned that, as a woman, my body would know what to do, and I had to get into agreement with this powerful process alongside genuine holistic care from midwives. The statistics for medical interventions during labour rise every year and is now around 60% in the UK. This suggests that, despite efforts to encourage women and give them choice, we are seeing a very different outcome.

I had to find a solution to this new picture of birth and wondered why in Bali I felt that birth would be an easy and joyful experience and, in the UK, it felt scary and potentially medical, because my body probably wouldn't know what to do? I had to find another way, so my quest for the truth began. I only had 3 months to figure it out!

I was lucky to attend a conference on birth from a holistic perspective, including leading scientists and thought leaders imparting amazing information. They all gave very positive messages about birth, which I found very helpful. The main message was this: surrender to the powerful energy of labour and try not to fear it, as this can help you through your birth.

However, this is easier said than done, especially as women and society have inherited the fear-based paradigm which is medical, painful, and a potential emergency. It starts with the language used by the well-meaning midwives or obstetricians, who explain the risks and offer all the available tests to see what might or could go wrong with our baby. This perspective instils a very subtle fear and lack of confidence in our body's inherent ability. (Once again, I experienced this recently with my sister's pregnancy). This encourages one to feel reliant on the professionals and the system. In addition, we are usually exposed to at least one birth horror story from women who carry around their unexpressed trauma. The ultimate legacy is the story of Eve, who would "give birth in great pain". It is, therefore, not surprising that many women automatically wish to opt out of the whole experience.

This encouraged me to start my own journey by healing my newly emerged fears of birth and other childhood traumas, including my own birth experience. I created lots of art which helped unlock buried feelings, and it was also fun. I read many books and explored *Source Process and Breathwork Therapy* (by Binnie A. Dansby), especially on mastering negative thought patterns and replacing them with positive affirmations. For example, instead of my newly emerged fear about the potential need for a caesarean, I changed my thoughts to: **"My body is safe no matter how I may be feeling"**. This became my mantra, and I believe this simple saying really made a significant difference. Luckily, this contrasting experience in Bali and the UK was the catalyst for the journey I've been on ever since.

I created a glass sculpture of my pregnant belly with the scan picture of my son printed on it, called "Life Before Birth to illustrate my deep feelings about pregnancy. It is easy to forget that, behind the belly of a pregnant woman there is a human being developing, taking shape, and creating its identity and uniqueness.

The heart starts to beat in the first few weeks after conception. The brain is building its neuropathways, and the cellular memory is storing data while the silent, invisible story forms within us. Creating a harmonious womb environment in pregnancy is desirable to enable the best outcome for the infant. Preparing for the birth is paramount. It is the transition from womb to world, which is a defining rite of passage, not only for the mother, but it is also the infant's first experience of life. I think we should treat this process with the sanctity it deserves.

During the latter part of my pregnancy, I had time to review my life and how my experiences had shaped me. My first and perhaps most obvious breakthrough was the realisation that every human being starts life inside a woman's body! I then discovered that this experience has an impact that stays with us throughout life, creating our first blueprint.

My journey revealed something really important: we need to hand the power back to women and encourage them to trust their own intuition and body wisdom. With this power, they can birth and parent their children and ask for what they want. This is where art therapy can be very powerful. There is a consensus that what women need during pregnancy and labour is the continuity of care by a known midwife, who is kind, gentle, and relaxed and trusts the deeper nature of the birth process. Our bodies are designed to give birth as our hormones trigger a dance between our body and our baby, so we can co-create life together. There is no need for constant interference. But, if for some reason a little extra help is needed, we have a competent medical system and technology close at hand. **Midwives are pivotal to the outcome.**

Another revelation was how feelings or past experiences are rarely acknowledged as having an influence on foetal development, birth, or a woman's health and wellbeing.

Birthing with medical intervention is increasing every year, suggesting that something is going on. The psychology of birth is missing.

Consider the messages given to pregnant women:
• It is safer to have your baby in hospital, which immediately suggests you can't be trusted to do it without a medical team standing by.
• There are countless tests you can have, making you immediately worry about something going wrong
• You're getting old and you are therefore at higher risk
• You're low risk or high risk. The process is fear based

We also do not honour the emotional/psychological experiences of women, such as:
• The impact of your environment and relationships during pregnancy (domestic violence often starts or increases during pregnancy)
• Previous birth stories (if you've already had a difficult birth, then this may influence your next pregnancy)
• You may have experienced pregnancy loss, which will certainly have an impact on your emotional well-being, especially in subsequent pregnancies.

The journey from conception to motherhood is the perfect time to start healing these emotional experiences, especially childhood trauma, and continue throughout life. There needs to be adequate support for women to get back in touch with their intuitive side, which can be achieved by exploring their non-verbal and unconscious psyche. Many different perspectives surround each woman's life, her circumstances, and her past, so one can never generalise or portray a one-size-fits-all situation.

However, if we re-establish a relationship with our deeper selves, with nature, and the spiritual or mystical and not just the physical and medical side of pregnancy, then birth might be less stressful for the mother and baby. Perhaps it is about finding a balance between science, technology, intuition, and nature. As an artist and art psychotherapist, I make parallel comparisons between the creative expression of art and birth; art is the physical representation of our unconscious world, and birth provides a bridge between the invisible and the visible. This is why I feel that art is a compatible way to explore our pregnancy and heal any fears.

I have been honoured to listen to thousands of birth stories, mostly painful experiences, told by women who carry this undigested experience around with them, waiting for it to be acknowledged. We also carry our own personal birth experience with us in our unconscious and cellular memory.

Witnessing a woman's journey through art therapy in a safe, nurturing space is one way to regenerate the current paradigm. I also think fathers need much more support, as they have their own journey and experience to be validated.

Finally, after three months of exploration, I got my head around the idea of a home birth and felt ready. On the 15th of January, 2000, I gave birth to a beautiful 9lb baby boy by candlelight in my living room, without any pain relief, cutting, tearing, or trauma. It was nothing like it's portrayed in the movies or on TV, which made me feel like I'd been lied to or that I had only been given one side of the story. For many, it is slow, gentle, quiet, and even pleasurable or orgasmic.

Birth is the most natural thing in the world and one of the most powerful rites of passage women can experience (if we want to have children). However, most of us have lost our intuitive inner compass. The more we cultivate a relationship with our body's wisdom and listen to its messages, the easier it will be to self-care, know our deepest desires, love and respect ourselves, and open up to the act of giving birth. I believe then that women will truly change the world.

Women are the birth keepers! We are responsible for bearing the next generation of this planet – with a man's help, of course! One of the benefits of giving birth at home is that there is much less interference. When my son was born, we had instant skin-to-skin contact, and when he woke up, he immediately breast fed. A secure attachment and bond were created from the first moment of life. There was no birth separation. If babies are immediately separated from their mothers at birth, it is very traumatic, and the longer the separation, the deeper the imprint. A newborn can experience it as a terrifying event that creates the foundation of a pattern on the primary blueprint of our lives. This embodied yet unconscious memory can show up in relationships throughout life, causing a real visceral fear of separation and other complications.

I am convinced that this gentle birth was all down to healing my fears and limiting beliefs in a creative, supportive, nurturing way so I could deeply trust myself and my body to birth outside the system. I was able to surrender to the unknown process, the chaos, the powerful, full-spectrum, energetic experience of birthing another human being!

I breast fed for two years, co-slept or had him in my room for quite some time, never let him cry himself to sleep, allowed him to express his feelings, and gave him as much love and attention as he required. I provided a positive continuum from conception to the present day.

My son is now an adult and is truly an amazing young man who entered the world in a peaceful, gentle, loving way. Whatever experiences came thereafter, his first moments of life gave him the strong message that life is safe, and he was very welcome and utterly loved.

I want all women to have this possibility whether you give birth at home, hospital, or birthing unit. We must change the current paradigm to integrate science/technology with the holistic mind, body, and spirit approach to bring about much-needed balance.

Women deserve to experience the power of birth and be supported and encouraged, not be traumatized by it. A more holistic, gentle, pleasurable approach to pregnancy and birth, with the right support from midwives and health visitors who are wise birth keepers, can gradually create global change. One could even go one step further and say that, in a wider context, healing ourselves and gently birthing human beings without trauma will help heal the earth, because a gentle birth can create a gentle earth and a better future for humanity.

(Disclaimer: I would like to acknowledge that the terms "woman," "women," and "mother" and the related pronouns have been used throughout this chapter. I respectfully recognise that some people who give birth may identify with another gender term.)

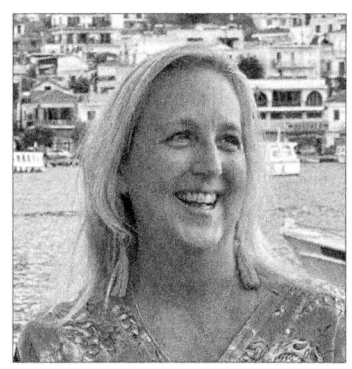 **Alex Florschutz, MA,** is a practicing artist, author of The Art of Birth – Empower Yourself for Conception, Pregnancy and Birth, Art Psychotherapist and exhibition curator and is currently Artist in Residence at University College London (UCL). Alex has studied perinatal/birth psychology for over 20 years, worked with pregnant women through art therapy, lectured at Middlesex University, given a speech in Parliament and created the Birthing a Better Future Art & Science Exhibition.

Please visit: www.zero2expo.com

Chapter 8

ANCIENT BALANCE OF
THE NEW HUMANITY

By Dale Allen

Sacred Vows Preceding Conception

"I want this experience with all my heart and soul.

I am willing to believe that we are co-creating Heaven on Earth.

I am willing to remember my True Nature, My Divinity.

I am willing to bring forth a Being of Light.

I recognize that this Being is arriving at precisely the right moment and in precisely the right package.

I am willing to recognize the Radiance of Her Being even before Her conception and through all the days that I carry Her growing body.

I am willing to support this Being in ways that will assist Him in staying "awake," that He may never need to fall into the sleep of forgetting His True Nature.

I am willing to do this by offering the same support to myself.

I am willing to accept all parts of this journey.
I see perfection in His physical form.

I see perfection in the contours of Her mind.

I see perfection in the gifts, talents, and insights He brings.

I see the perfection of Her own pace and unique unfolding.

I am willing to hold the vision that love is possible at all times, on every level, and in every experience.

I am willing. I am willing. I am willing.

May every child be regarded as the Holy One he or she is, as we all commit to embracing a thriving human family and planet. Heaven is here and now, on Earth."

These are the words that came to me years ago, just prior to the conception of my daughter. I was in a centuries-old cathedral in Switzerland, looking at a beautiful painting of Mary and Jesus. Tears were streaming down my face. After a series of miscarriages and the deep heartbreak surrounding them, I had been praying fervently for a child to successfully arrive. At that time, I was also in the wake of having let go of the career path that I had been on, one I was very invested in, and this was a disappointing loss. It was a time of void. It was a time of sorrow. I had witnessed the tumbling down of the structure of my core beliefs and my faith in life.

During that period, I started writing poetry as a way to access my deeper feelings, and I noticed a new voice whispering up from the depths of my being. It was feminine. This was new to me.

Mother Soil

The black night of the soul
The great black void
Is where with bare hands
I till and turn
Rich Mother soil
Sacred emptiness
The very place of the inception
of the seed of infinite possibility

During this period, the term "Goddess" kept crossing my path, and I noticed that I didn't like it. It felt uncomfortable and unnecessary. I didn't like the way it brought gender into any discussion of the divine. For me, if I were to use the term "God," it would be to describe something beyond gender – the energy behind all things, Supreme Love, the Creator, complete and becoming at the same time. Since I didn't see any gender imbalance in my view at the time, I was surprised at how much I resisted the term "Goddess." As a person in a female body, I thought perhaps I should investigate these feelings. Indeed, it was my very resistance to the term that caused me to go headlong into it. I studied the work of historians, anthropologists, archaeologists, psychologists, poets, artists, and philosophers. The more I persisted in my studies of the sacred feminine, the more I realized just how deeply embedded male monotheism had been in my psyche. Even though we may hold that the divine is beyond gender, whether we are agnostic or atheist, we are affected by the male monotheistic cultures in which we live.

This journey into the sacred feminine was profoundly transformative for me and was helpful to me in my sorrow surrounding my fertility. I had a revelation that my fertility could take the form of any kind of creativity, and I knew it would be healthy to align with the joy and energy of the create principle. I began saying to myself, "I am the most fertile woman on the planet!" (Not compared to anyone else, just exuberantly declaring this energy for myself.)

I remembered what it felt like to be a girl, just creating because I felt like it. As a girl, I didn't ask, "How can I market this? Am I good enough to make this? How can I make this a business? Will I succeed?" I just created because creativity feels good. And so, harnessing my girl-self exuberance, I decided to write a play. I proceeded in the spirit of fun and abandon, like my 11-year-old self would have. I decided to write a play about the Goddess. How could I not share Her? I had found my journey into the sacred feminine to be so healing, I simply had to share it.

As I reflect on it all now, I can't help but see a kind of divine orchestration. In the pain of my experience, the disappointment in my career path, the sorrow of miscarriages – in the great black void – the sacred feminine entered for me. Furthermore, it has shaped my life, work and focus since then, and has played a huge part in my motherhood. That reflection leaves me awestruck and humbled. It reminds me that if we can just step back far enough in our perspective, we often see that somehow, beauty on a Soul-level is unfolding.

This is what began my career in sharing the sacred feminine. It started with writing, producing, directing, and performing in a successful musical production in Westport, Connecticut, with a cast of seven women of different ages, shapes, sizes, and colors. This first theatrical production showed me how hungry women and men are for positive and powerful images of the feminine – for the sacred feminine. It showed me how necessary it is for women and men to know "HERstory," the story that isn't told. Women do not know the collective wounds they carry nor the impact these wounds have on their lives. The response to the play showed me the need for this work. After success in Connecticut, I was beginning to organize a production at a theater in New York, when I learned I was pregnant! And this time, I experienced the bliss of a great round belly and the birth of my daughter!

I am grateful that my pregnancy came after I had been saturated in exquisite images of the Goddess, often depicted with her round belly. I was aligned with the Mother of All Things who births all of creation and deeply loves and nurtures all that She creates. I reveled in roundness! I delighted in being so tuned in to the Being whose body was taking shape in my womb and whose Spirit was the vastness of the Universe, along with mine. I was in constant communion with this Being, and together, we presided over the development of the tiny new physical body within me.

In my studies of the sacred feminine and in my play, I had explored contemporary and historical cultures that venerate a female creator, wherein gestation and birth are celebrated, natural, and empowering. The womb, the darkness, and the void are sacred. The Goddess creates with her female body. Life develops in Her womb and arrives though the birth canal. The Mother loves and nurtures her creation. Beautiful art and artifacts of Goddess cultures depict peace and centeredness during pregnancy as the Goddess gestates life. The male monotheistic cultures that appeared with the emergence of alphabetic literacy brought new creation myths, and they rejected all knowledge of female birthing. New Sky Gods did amazing new things like eject life through their foreheads. Or, the new Sky Gods fought fearsome battles, killing great serpents and sea snakes (representations of the Goddess) to gain control of the universe. Creation became an abstraction of the mind, word, or will through acts of violence. The rise of alphabetic literacy and male monotheism brought hierarchy and gender imbalance to the human experience. Women and all things feminine became suspect and the downfall of the pious man. The female body was dangerous, no longer sacred. Women, rather than feeling the power and blessing of the Goddess during pregnancy and birth, instead were deeply influenced by new cultural thoughtforms, for example: "I will greatly multiply thy sorrows and thy conceptions, in pain shalt thou bring forth children…" (Genesis 3:16) In retrospect, I am grateful that I had explored and shared all this – and so much more – in the period before my own pregnancy and birth experience.

My daughter was born into a home that had beautiful Goddess energy and celebration of the feminine. It was – and is – a home of magic, wonder, play, imagination, and creativity. I decided to turn my musical production into a one-woman show, which I could more easily manage with my motherhood. I began touring my show by booking it, performing, and coming right back home to my family. My own mother came with me on some of these performances, handling the technical aspects of the show. I toured the piece for the next 15 years.

It is powerful to realize at this point how my daughter arrived after I came to embrace the Feminine Face of the Divine. I had come to see the impact of male monotheism in my life, not by looking directly at male monotheism, but by turning my attention toward the awkwardness of the feminine pronouns for the divine. For me, the awkwardness has melted away. Feedback from scores of audiences lets me know that my sharing the sacred feminine in the way I do has been, and continues to be, healing for others. Invigorating the feminine energy within to create a balance with the masculine energy within is something we all benefit from: men, women, LGBTQIA2+ persons – everyone. And this in turn balances our cultures and our world.

Our Mother

Our Mother who art within us
Each breath brings us to you.
Thy wisdom come,
Thy will be done as we honor your presence within us.
You give us this day all that we need.
Your bounty calls us to give and receive

all that is loving and pleasurable.
You are the courage that moves us to be true to ourselves and we act with grace and power.
We relax into your cycles of birth, death, and renewal.
Out of the womb, the darkness, the void,
comes new life.
For you are the Mother of All Things.
Your body is the Sacred Earth and our bodies.
Your love nurtures us and unites us all.
Now and forever more.

We have all incarnated in precise and perfect timing for this moment on the planet, and we can see that we are at a critical point. All my life, I have watched two vast waves of energy coming toward each other: fear and love. Fear is the main broadcast we hear and see from our news sources, and there are very real concerns. Indeed, the Earth's health needs our protection. Technologies like smart phones, virtual reality, artificial intelligence, deep fakes, and social media challenge the very essence of being a human with our own face, voice, name, and reputation. We are being reduced to a swipe left or right, an image that we or others can easily manipulate. Global powers have weapons now that are incomprehensibly powerful and insidious. It is overwhelming. However, here we are, in perfect timing. There are many of us on this Earth who are holding the grid, tending our thoughts, dedicating our offerings for a world of peace and balance. And there is still a long line of Souls wanting to get here to Earth. These Souls are counting on us.

We each have our part to play and gifts to offer. I am still called to share the sacred feminine, and so I do. It's not about religion for me, and I often present the material through the lens of the archetypes, as offered by Carl Jung, to steer clear of religion. I do not assert any particular gender of the deity, nor the existence thereof. These notions can create division and bog us down. What matters is Life, now. Love, now. And co-creating a world wherein every child is seen as the Holy Child they are.

I am interested in the progression of human consciousness. I'm interested in creating a global community and a way to share this precious earth. I'm interested in finding what unites us, our common history before the rise of the world's religions. I am interested in the historical evolutionary development of the human species, with a balance of masculine and feminine, and a balance of the right and left hemispheres of our brains, as designed before the left-brain dominance we know so well.

Just across the corpus collosum in each of our brains, from the left to the right hemisphere, is the presence, empathy, and understanding of our right brains – the "feminine gatherer-nurturer" side. We were designed with a balance of both hemispheres and a balance of both masculine and feminine energy. The imbalance we face arose fairly recently in the big scheme of things, beginning with alphabetic literacy. But 90% of our human history precedes our written history. We can look at historical and contemporary cultures of balance to see pieces of what is possible for us today and as we birth the new humanity. Thankfully, The Mother has left a Memory in us all.

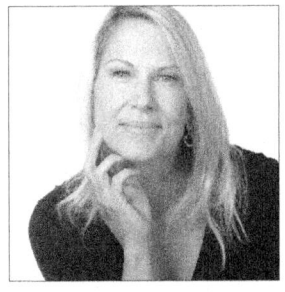

Dale Allen is a veteran of corporate, commercial, and creative communications with hundreds of voice-over, on-camera, theater, and keynote engagements. She has brought her talents to scores of audiences across the U.S. and Canada and from Kauai to Dubai and the United Nations. With the energy of "a Cape Canaveral lift-off," she thoroughly engages and inspires her audience, which ranges from highly educated corporate leaders to teenage girls seeking their place in the world.

www.thecore.space
www.inourrightminds.net

Chapter 9

A MIDWIFE'S PLEA

By Karima Hakimi

I was born in Afghanistan. On that day, I had not even opened my eyes to see my mother's beautiful face. As a newborn, I was far from realizing what destiny had in store for me. I was left alone in a corner of this country where being a girl is a crime in itself. My mother had just died from postpartum hemorrhage. She would have been my only protector, but she was gone.

My father abandoned me, as was his right in this country, not taking any responsibility for my upbringing. Instead, he relieved himself of the burden and never showed up. If I had been a boy, I may have had the chance to be hugged by him.

It is considered normal for my father to remarry and never come to see me. Instead, he gave me immediately to a couple who had no children.

Although my adoptive parents were both illiterate, they were good people. It was by chance one day that my true story came to light. I was seven years old when I heard from my neighbors that, in fact, my mum and dad were not my real parents. I was in shock and wanted to know my origins.

It was common where I grew up for women to be treated like used objects. I was very fortunate to have escaped the fate of many girls my age. They are considered "property" that can be exchanged for money or goods. This may seem unreal, but it's the sad and appalling reality. I would see my friends who were between 9 and 12 years old forced to marry Taliban soldiers. By doing so, they thought they would keep their families safe. A young girl in the family had to be sacrificed. Countless little girls disappeared, and no one ever heard anything from them again, at least while they were alive.

I was hardworking, and as I grew up I became very interested in education. I was always studying at night by candlelight and was considered to be an excellent student. Early in life I became passionate about aviation and desperately wanted to become a pilot. I studied hard to make this dream come true.

However, when my first menstrual period began, my thoughts went to my biological mother. I had learnt that she had bled to death, and upon seeing my own bleeding, I thought that this was my mother bleeding to death. I was terrified and had no one to talk to about my painful birth wound that was surfacing in my mind. This was a decisive moment. Instead of becoming a pilot, I would become a midwife. I wanted to save the lives of mothers and prevent other children from growing up as I did. Perhaps I could even change the way mothers are treated.

In addition to years of war, poverty, and illiteracy, the people of Afghanistan witness horrific events. Regularly people are burned alive, thrown in wells, and even have their ears and noses cut off. This especially happens to women. It is quite clear that our first major problem is that we, the people, are in a country at war where, unfortunately, most of the victims are civilians. The second major problem in Afghanistan is the male domination through which women are the victims.

For decades, these women have been sacrificed. It is not unusual for us to hear about someone's ears and nose being cut off in Herat, someone who was stoned to death and later burned in Kabul, someone who was raped by his father in Baghlan, or someone whose body was found in a barrel in Kabul. We always knew that they were women. Away from the eyes of the mass media and even from the eyes of families, these women are becoming victims, day by day. You can imagine the trauma, fear, and anxiety that we live with.

In this country, women do not yet have an independent legal identity. They are still defined as men. For example, naming and specifying a woman's name is taboo. A woman here, in the best of cases, is still a man's sister, a man's mother, and a man's wife. If women are respected or given a right, it is for them to be sisters and mothers in cohabitation and not as a free, independent human being.

Educated and seemingly intelligent Afghan men are still proudly chanting that they give women in their families the right to work and study. This means that even the very low percentage of our society is educated and intelligent. They consider themselves the owners of the rights of women in their families and do not look at women as independent legal entities who own their own rights. It is common for women to be treated even worse by illiterate men.

One may ask why no one defends their rights and opposes these immoral demands. The answer is clear to everyone. Anyone who tries to oppose them pays the price of even greater sacrifices. This hell on earth shouldn't exist, but how can we change it? This torment became so intense that I wanted badly to leave this country.

When I was 11 years old and in sixth grade at school, the Taliban closed the schools to girls. No girl had the right to education, and women were forbidden to work outside the home. I remember well that the Taliban had built their own checkpoint at the school, and every time I passed by the school walls, I wished the classroom bell would ring again. After two years, I was allowed back to school again. I finally graduated but with great difficulty. I took the university entrance exam and entered the Kabul Institute of Health Sciences.

I was studying in a girls' dormitory in Kabul when I heard that my father had a stroke. He could not speak, and his right arm and leg could not move properly. The cold nights in the dormitory were unbearable. We did not even have a warm place where we could sleep. My body became weak with this stress and the extremely poor food.

It became apparent that I had to accept the advances of one of my suitors. I needed someone to support me. I met Javid, who seemed like a good boy and someone I could trust. He told me that he would never interfere with my studies and work in the community.

Parental consent is necessary to marry in Afghanistan. If the parents were happy, we had the right to live together. If the parents were dissatisfied, we had no right to marry. Fortunately, my marriage was not like this. Javid and I had seen each other and reached an agreement for our families to talk to each other. However, my marriage ended up with the dissatisfaction of my adoptive mother. Even though I had not known the love of my real mother, I loved her like my mother and perhaps even more. Unfortunately, she did not think I did. For years her behavior tortured me emotionally after my marriage. She was outraged. How could I possibly give myself the right to marry someone she was dissatisfied with?

Now, independent from my parents and married, I finally completed my studies and received my diploma in midwifery. My first job was in the remote and mountainous province of Daikundi. Maternal mortality was high, and there was still a shortage of doctors and midwives. I worked there for several months and later returned to Kabul and worked at Esteghlal Hospital. I helped a lot of mothers ease their pain during labor. With a smile and much satisfaction, I put many babies in the loving arms of their mothers.

Due to my father's health, I returned to Baghlan, where I became a midwifery instructor. For four years I trained many young women in midwifery so that they could take care of the mothers during childbirth in the remote villages. I too travelled to these villages to supervise and support health centers and midwives provide quality health services. I continued my studies pursuing health and legal education so that I could inform women in the villages about their reproductive and gender rights.

I continually advised them that it is not good for a mother and her child's health if she marries at a very young age and counseled them to leave adequate spacing between children. Women need to know about their gender rights so they will not be misled. Even though I did not travel alone without my husband, which was required, my activities were often condemned.

In Afghanistan, pregnancy and motherhood are the most difficult stages of life for women. Even though I enjoyed becoming a mother, during my pregnancy, according to family customs and traditions, I had to do all the housework myself. In addition, I had to deal with all the problems and take care of the whole family. I only had twenty days off after giving birth, even though I was a midwife, and had to return to work with my 20-day-old baby.

Every Afghan woman's life is like a dry leaf, dried and fragile with surrender. It comes with turmoil, and its destiny is turbulent. This feeling gripped me years ago and still does. But my resolve is to be strong, hopeful, and hardworking. I knew I had to leave Afghanistan for the safety of my life and the future of my children.

One day we found a way to escape from this hell. With little knowledge of the outside world, we abandoned everything and fled. All we wanted was to go to a place without unnecessary war and no sacrifices for the useless achievements of others. It took several months of hardship and unhappiness until, in August 2017, we finally arrived in Jakarta, Indonesia.

We were very happy to have finally overcome the hardships and conflicts of the war and looked forward to living in a peaceful environment. Once again, our destiny turned. I was two months pregnant when we arrived in Indonesia with my two sons, my husband, and my mother. After registering with UNHCR Indonesia, we asked for asylum. They refused, saying that they had no shelter for refugees and no budget, so we had to sleep on the street for a week. The immigration police imprisoned us.

In prison, we found ourselves in the same cell as drug traffickers. My family and I were locked in a small room for four months. The room didn't even have a small window to see if it was day or night. We were only allowed to spend two hours in the sun once a week. Life in Indonesia was becoming another nightmare. It has now been almost five years since we have been living here as refugees. My family and I are still imprisoned in a camp, and our activities are limited.

We have no right to work, no right to education, no right to travel from one city to another, and no right to education for our children. We do not even have the right to have a bank account and buy a SIM card. Refugees in Indonesia do not have access to even the most basic human rights. Some refugees even call Indonesia "The Green Hell." Once again, we know this is not the way to live. We are constantly having to make many changes in ourselves and to adapt and improve our way of thinking, our way of life, and our beliefs.

The realization of a girl's dreams begins with the trust and support of their families. The most successful are those who have this support and pursue their dreams with a strong belief. My heart yearns for women everywhere to be free and equal to men, treated with dignity and empowerment to let go of their fears and limitations.

Women, and especially mothers, have an amazing job to do. It is important that they begin educating their babies in the womb, teaching them that brothers and sisters are equal and celebrating the unique characteristics of each gender.

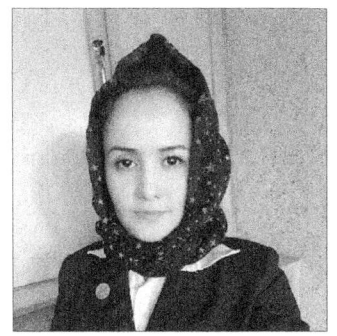 **Karima Hakimi** is an Afghan midwife and trainer. A mother of four, she and her family fled the harsh conditions of her homeland and the tremendous gender inequalities. She currently lives in appalling conditions in a refugee camp in Jakarta, Indonesia. Karima is an advocate for gender equality, human rights, and dignity and speaks four languages fluently. She is seeking asylum in a country where her family can blossom and she can serve birthing mothers.

Chapter 10

MUMS IN SLUMS

By Moffat Osoro

How do you find your life purpose and path? Life is beautiful and crafted for every form of life. We are all partakers and champions of something bigger, better, and desirable for the world. How do we pursue our purpose, our vocation, and our calling? We need to look at the big picture of humanity. There is no real life without humanity at its core. To be humane is to identify oneself as a responsible being who has a role to play in order to make life better, not just for oneself, but also for all creatures on the planet.

I was born in the 1980s in Kisii, Nyanza region, Kenya, in East Africa. I was the sixth of my parents' eight children. I didn't have an easy childhood. Most of the time, we were a happy family, but the challenges of poverty were constant. I went to school early, which explains my high school graduation at a young age. My best memories are of the beautiful Kisii highlands and being in a large family that gave me love, security, and a sense of belonging. I was strong and tough. If other children insulted me, I would have my own way to get them to pay for it. In grade three, two boys, including my desk mate, started bullying me. I crafted a plan to punish them: I looked for canes and soaked them in salt for several days. On the last day of school, I caned the two bullies mercilessly before rushing back home.

I was not born to just stand for myself but for the vulnerable as well. Some kids had taken advantage of me because I was young and tiny, but I didn't give in. This gave me the necessary confidence and stamina to keep helping people in difficulty. I still do it today.

I lived very tough times. To protect their privacy, I won't say much about my family, but the challenges we met taught me to stand up for myself and others. The trials and experience accumulated earlier gave me the energy to start the Fremo clinic project.

I had been rejected many times when seeking medical care, and I knew that I had to find a solution. This sparked my dream of better medical practices, resulting in a better world.

Accessing medical care in Kenya is a challenge due to poverty, lack of skilled providers, and the need of many licenses to practice. Establishing a medical facility in these conditions didn't feel like a walk in the park.

My story, like many others, is about finding my place, being at peace with it, and making it shine.

I soon moved to the Kawangware community. It was dirty, insecure, congested, and lacking the most basic social amenities. In the countryside where I grew up, it is easy to find a place to get treated. They call it a dispensary. But in a city like Kawangware, it can be very hard. Small chemists and roadside clinics are mushrooming all over the place. They all claim to treat, but nothing is less true.

I got sick with what would later be diagnosed as typhoid. I was struggling to cope with the many treatments I received from the community clinics, but it was in vain. At the same time, my brother Fred was becoming a clinical doctor. I invited him to treat me and made a commitment that when I got better, I would work to change these poor medical conditions.

I did get cured, and a few months later, my dream started concretizing. My frustration, associated with a strong desire to make it better, started to bear fruit. The process was long and difficult, as we needed a proper design and a skilled professional team. Nevertheless, a few years later, the Fremo clinic was born and working.

Soon after the opening of our medical center, my wife finally got pregnant. Due to her high blood pressure, we couldn't keep her at Fremo for the birth. She was transferred to a government referral hospital. This resulted in mistreatment and frustration. My wife was admitted, but I was sent away. She was supposed to be induced, but they did almost nothing for two days. During the delivery, she was left with other birthing mothers, all in labour, on the floor in the same room, with hardly any support. They were struggling to cope with the labor pains with no caregiver or supporting companion by their side.

This was my wake-up call to change the whole setup and create a hospital that would practice, inculcate, and facilitate care with uncompromising compassion, kindness, love, gentleness, and social justice. As a result, I am delighted to say that my next two kids were welcomed in this world in a haven of love and kindness, in my presence, with a team of facilitators acting with the sweetness that brings joy, laughter, and beautiful tears to the eyes of birthing families.

Mother Empowerment
When I met Vicki Chan, a passionate, compassionate, and humanitarian being, it felt like the universe had put us together for a purpose. Vicki brought the skills that guided and rekindled the whole journey of birth. She was driven by the faith that her role as a midwife was to make every woman smile, feel dignified, and step out of maternity with no trauma, feeling loved and empowered to build a beautiful world for herself, her baby, and her family.

The agony and distress I had experienced during the birth of our first child, Frank, should never happen to another human being.

Who am I, and what makes me so passionate about birth? In my culture, no stage of the human life is treasured as much as birth. The pregnant woman is adored, respected, and treated with love, honor, and all the support she needs. We naturally love our mothers because, when birth is respected and properly facilitated, the bond with others is magnified. If you come close to a birth room and hear the cry of a newborn, you are listening to the voice of an angel. You've just witnessed the beginning of life.

If you've been blessed with taking part in childbearing and raising, you know what it means to be completely transformed. The love babies bring to the planet is so magical that everything in the universe seems to celebrate their arrival.

I was brought up in rural Kenya, and I raised my three kids in Nairobi. I can say that being part of birth and parenthood is the most important part of my life. As a professional psychologist, I can testify that the hundreds of cases I have been involved in are the result of lack of love often associated with violence during pregnancy, childbirth, growth, and development.

Most trauma originates from a missed opportunity to provide support when it's most needed. There couldn't be a better platform to avoid this than a place where mothers are encouraged to love their unborn baby, to birth in love, and to be provided with all the care and love the world needs to resolve today's turmoil.

The Care at Fremo Birth Centre
Fremo Birth Centre offers personalized antenatal care in which each woman is attended in a focused model of care by a midwife. All of her pregnancy needs are listened to and addressed informatively. Expectant mothers are encouraged to

be accompanied by their partner. They are reminded to eat and drink healthily, sleep under mosquito-treated nets, and come for regular appointments. They are advised to save for maternal care costs. We also remind them to take frequently required medicines, prophylaxis, and supplements.

Accessibility: The hospital and midwives can be accessed 24/7. This encourages women to seek help when they face challenges or encounter danger at home. Our appointed taxi is available in case a mother needs transport to the facility in the odd hours of the night.

Informed Choice: This is to help parents to educate themselves and learn about pregnancy, its challenges and dangers, as well as their caregivers.

Prenatal Visits and Follow-Up: Check up on enrollment, and during monthly visits, we make sure that mother and baby are coping and healthy. Those who require medical care receive it. Should the mothers need supplements, they are provided them. Preventive measures are discussed, and necessary interventions are provided.

Choice and dignity: We believe women should be the leaders of their care. They are human beings. They have rights, desires, and preferences. This should be recognized, respected, and acted upon accordingly.

Love, compassion, social justice, and community support are the pillars of totally functional and appreciative care. We have come to realize that language and communication should be at the center of all care. In many places, the language is vulgar and the communication patronizing. This should never happen! Autonomy and family support: Women are free to choose who they want in the birthing room. They can birth in the position in which they feel the most comfortable. They experience their labor the way they want and are invited to bring along the close ones they wish. We also advise them to eat and drink during labor.

Skin-to-skin care after birth is encouraged to enable mother and baby bonding. The team knows that mother and baby should never be separated from each other at birth. Breastfeeding is initiated during the first hour. We also delay cord clamping and baby weighing.

Mother and baby are allowed to stay for some time in the birth room so that they can rest, bond, and breastfeed. They are not rushed into postnatal care.

Prenatal care: We encourage love and self-care. A woman who is loved and willingly taking care of herself and her baby is an emancipated human being. In self-care, she gets to know herself, her weaknesses, and her strengths. With the right information, the decisions made during the journey to birth and motherhood are the best possible. We emphasize that women coming for follow-up will receive full support. And they do!

Postnatal Outreach
I initiated this program in 2012 at the Fremo Medical and Birth Centre. We were worried about the many challenges young mothers and babies faced at home.

The first question we asked patients was whether their home conditions where conducive to baby care after discharge. Most women portrayed humble background and facilities. It was our responsibility to visit them at home and audit the environment in order to evaluate how easy it would be for mother and baby to thrive, so we went on with the plan.

When discharged, mothers are asked to give permission to our outreach team to visit them within 24 or 48 hours. All contact information is noted, including their physical address.

On the announced day, a midwife takes the postnatal files and calls to inform the mother of the imminent follow-up. The driver and midwife go from house to house within the neighborhood. Mother and baby are checked and examined. Any deviation from normal postpartum is immediately addressed. Issues of lack of breastmilk, jaundice, abdominal pains, exhaustion, cord cleaning, and medication are discussed in detail. Concerns are brought back to the center for doctor's review and treatment. If the case is beyond the center's expertise, the person is referred to a specialist.

High-risk mothers with noticeable health challenges are either admitted at the centre or transferred to the National referral hospital. The high-risk cases may include mothers who are diabetic, hypertensive, or have chronic heart and congenital deformities.

If further management is required, our team is involved in the referral procedure until transfer and admission at the hospital. Our midwives are involved in the entire process.

Once the baby and mother have stabilized, they are discharged to go back home with the help of the hospital van. The outreach program is free at the client's home.

The main challenges occur when mothers refuse to give permission for treatment and come up with complications within a few hours or days. Also, some would allow our team in their homes but refuse to come back to the clinic if a health issue is discovered. The main reason seems to be that some people don't like to re-live any hospital experience after they have been discharged.

Mother's Day
This is a very important day of the interaction and scorecard of our clinic. Mothers who gave birth at the center are invited to share and celebrate the care they received. They introduce themselves and have the opportunity to talk about their

experience, their difficulties in labor, their evaluation of the team performance, and what could have been done better. They receive an anonymous questionnaire so that they don't feel they will be reprimanded later for describing a negative experience. It is also the occasion to discuss child welfare clinics, family planning, parenting and parenthood, clinical dangers at home for babies, breastfeeding, and HIV, among other topics.

Family Planning
All non-surgical family planning methods are available to all reproductive mothers. Pills, injectables, condoms, and long-term family planning methods are accessible and given.

Prevention of Mother-To-Child Transmission (PMTCT)
Mother and child care and treatment are provided for HIV positive mothers and their babies. Testing, treatment, and care are provided for free in partnership with the government and local NGOs.

Our nutrition department is well established, too. It looks after the nutritional challenges of mothers and malnourished children. It also supports HIV-infected mothers, providing them with supplements at no cost. We visit them at home in order to give them the best possible assistance and create a strong rapport with their caregiver and the center.

Over the years, the Fremo Clinic has gained such a reputation that some wealthy women choose to deliver their babies in a center initially created to help the poorest. The language of love knows no financial borders, and we are demonstrating every day that no sophisticated machinery could ever replace love and compassion in the great endeavor of Birthing the New Humanity.

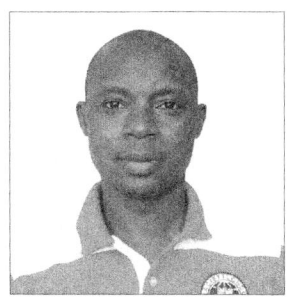 **Moffat Osoro** is a Kenyan psychologist who lives in Nairobi. In 2009, with practically no money, he created the Fremo medical facility to offer affordable quality medical care to the people of Kawangware, informal settlement. This was a big task, as he had no medical background at the time. 13 years later, the center is attracting global attention for its high quality, gentle assistance to families and women seeking compassionate maternal care.

Chapter 11

CRUCIBLES

By Adela Barcia

I took my very first step on the path to becoming a psychotherapist when I was five. One day in kindergarten, I experienced empathic knowing for the first time. I could feel what little Charles was feeling across the playground during recess and remember saying to myself, "Someone should help him, he hurts inside." In that moment, I hurt inside, too, which is how I recognized his pain.

My loving parents were puzzled as to why it was so hard for me to go to school. Each morning when my mother would leave me, I would cry inconsolably. My separation anxiety overrode any desire to play or learn. However, given my birth experience, it makes perfect sense. I was the baby my mother pleaded with the nurse to comfort after a long night of hearing me scream and cry in the nursery just down the hall, not knowing I was hers. I know the truth of birth trauma and attachment ruptures in my own body. They left a deep imprint that colored my childhood and parts of my adult life until I finally released the last vestiges in a somatic process, in Breathwork.

During my first Breath session, I had an extraordinary experience. I did not realize there was any residue of my birth imprint left to heal, but this is where the Breath took me. First, I went through the terror and the tears until they were spent from my body. Then I found myself in the birth canal, moving toward the light, and I was born. I saw my mother's face, but this time she stayed with me. Her eyes looked back at me, full of love.

Then, other eyes appeared until all I could see were eyes – they were the eyes of every person that had ever loved me, holding me with love. The efficiency of my own being knowing exactly where I needed to go, creating the somatic release and then the healing experience amazed me. Naturally, after this powerful transformative experience, I trained to become a Breathworker.

I have been a practicing psychotherapist for more than four decades. Over time, I learned a great deal about what it takes for people to change internally and then to make different decisions. Watching thousands of people up close as they navigated their most tender internal territories, I acquired a rich education in human nature, both dark and light, and learned what contributes to a disposition toward one or the other. I have had a panoramic view of what enables people to thrive and what hampers and impedes them. My clients' experiences, as well as my own, have given me a comprehensive understanding of trauma, how to prevent it, and how to heal it. Recently, I have been contemplating how to apply what I've observed in individuals to the collective culture.

There are many complex reasons why trauma colors so much of our modern world. From a pre- and perinatal perspective, the fact that many people begin their lives in trauma must be identified as one of the cornerstone causes. This makes what happens at birth both a potent variable to address and a readily available point of intervention.

Medicalized birth practices have profoundly disrupted the perfect system nature had evolved for birthing babies disposed to thrive. Consequently, in most developed countries, traumatic birth and incomplete attachment with the mother are very often human beings' first experiences in life. We now know that many lifelong patterns and dispositions are set in both our neurobiology and our psyches from prebirth through the end of the prime attachment phase at age five. Consider how differently we might face and integrate life's ongoing challenges if those earliest experiences of the world unfolded as they were meant to and the very young felt safe and loved rather than stressed and afraid. Surprisingly, not long after the somatic release of the last layer of my birth trauma, I noticed that I felt much more at ease when giving a talk or presentation. Perhaps my previous reluctance to use my voice was connected in some way to what had imprinted in my newborn self when I cried and screamed, and nobody came.

In my early thirties, I had a series of compelling experiences that catapulted me into a different way of perceiving the world. It was the beginning of my spiritual awakening and despite some power invitations, I resisted. What finally impelled me into deep metaphysical inquiry and a profound shift in my world view, also ultimately led to my work in pre- and perinatal health and psychology – my most passionate specialty for over 30 years.

I had completed an intensive training program in Eriksonian hypnotherapy and began doing in-depth work in this modality with my clients. It seemed like magic to be able to ask the unconscious mind for answers and to receive such rich responses. In trance, I would ask a client to return to the first time they had ever experienced the troubling feeling that they wished to shed. What happened was unexpected: they would often narrate experiences that happened in the womb, or at their birth, and sometimes they would recount their conception! I was stunned, and I wanted proof. Time after time, when my clients would question their mother or father about what they had remembered in trance, they would receive validation. How could they have formed memories when there was little or no brain development, much less remember their conception?

Within the paradigm that had informed how I saw the world, there was no way to explain or understand what my clients were reporting. Prenatal memories require that consciousness exist independent of our physicality, and this was not something that I believed. After many more irrefutable experiences, I finally yielded, and my personal cosmology eventually shifted from physical materialism to quantum mechanics.

When I began to work with birth, I was fascinated to experience the same sacred space I had discovered during my years working with AIDS patients and death and dying. It made sense – after all, birth and death are the bookends of the life experience. It was a rarefied space that seemed outside of the ordinary more linear world, where exponential healing would happen. I developed a model for intergenerational healing during pregnancy, culminating in empowered birth. It was joyful work with many expectant Mamas over the years. I loved it!

The next phase of my development came from outside of my psycho/spiritual framework. I was invited to an event that introduced me to the indigenous world. I met Elders from all over the world and spent the next few years attending gatherings and absorbing the teachings of those who had grown up in the old ways. I came to embrace Mother Earth with new respect and to consider all beings my relatives. I was introduced to ceremony, to the drum that opens the heart, and to the wisdom of first nations' values and practices. These experiences gently and often joyfully transformed me. I began to experience a new lightness of being as I felt a sense of my place within the web of life and the easing of an individualism I had not known was a burden. As I began to feel the Earth herself as a living being that I loved, I also felt a new responsibility to care for her that I could not ignore.

Both our internal and social systems have become increasingly out of balance. It's hard to fathom how we humans can continue to make choices that push us closer to an irreversible environmental tipping point. This dangerous degree of denial demonstrates characteristics of a trauma reaction; being numb and immobilized in the face of a real threat is a fight/flight/freeze reaction. When we look at many of our social ills through the trauma lens, many causal factors suddenly come into sharp relief.

In our industrialized and now technocratic modern life, so many of the structures and systems that kept us connected to valuable aspects of our humanity have fallen away. Foremost among these is having a sense of belonging to something outside of ourselves. When we stopped evolving, we belonged to a tribe of other humans and to the land. Even after we became urbanized, we still belonged to extended family and to communities. Within both of these were expectations and roles that we understood and could fulfil, and this organized and grounded a sense of self and value. We felt connected, and because we cared about one another, this added a layer of coherence to our common human experience. We belonged to neighborhoods in which we formed life-long relationships with people of all ages and stages of life that we could learn from organically as we navigated those stages ourselves. So few people enjoy these vital bonds in their lives anymore. What we belong to and what belongs to us, what we are attached to, we tend to love and therefore want to care for.

I believe we are collectively in a kind of generalized attachment rupture. I see this as one of the causes of the profound lack of empathy that has become endemic in modern societies and that has made such large numbers of people indifferent to suffering. Many individuals in our culture are so self-absorbed that they disregard whatever does not benefit them directly, a dangerous trait in those with great wealth and power. One could say that we are in a crisis caused by a disruption in our ability to love.

I am often asked what my hope for the future of our world is based on. It is based on faith; on the way I see and understand life. As I look back, my most deeply formative experiences were not so much those that developed my mind and honed my skills, but those that served as the fertile terrain for my unfolding consciousness. I believe that life is an expression of a unified energy field, a Oneness. A change in the consciousness of individuals will be mirrored in the changing consciousness of the collective. I believe in the fundamental goodness of most people and have witnessed enough miracles to know the tremendous power of love. I genuinely believe in the possibility of global transformation, that humanity can rise to this challenge. Having real hope gives me a platform to be among the voices that provide a way forward. Today, I will keep my eye on the light, even though to many it seems like a mere glimmer.

We have been poor stewards of our planetary home, and Mother Earth is letting us know. The trajectory of global warming urgently needs a course correction. This requires an exponential change in the consciousness of enough people to reach a tipping point in human consciousness before we reach an environmental one. Still, we need only look at what Greta Thunberg has done to know that some truly gifted leaders might be sufficient to catalyze the necessary energy. When enough people rise up, even stable socio/political systems change. We have seen it happen before.

I will close with one last story: In 2013, I went to India for the first time for a retreat with Julie and Francois Gerland. A few of us gathered in the Southern Himalayas at a retreat center that Julie had intuitively selected. We went during the Navratri festival time to ask for the blessing of the Divine Mother while we conceived the project we would internally gestate until the new year, nine months away. The project was Birthing The New Humanity. We were staying only a kilometer away from the venue where I was registered to attend my first International Breathwork Foundation Congress – quite the coincidence! I returned to India three more times that year and had a bounty of experiences that confirmed my quantum theory perspective on the nature of the world.

In order to dedicate myself to the potential contribution I would make at this threshold, in 2019 I radically changed my life. I shifted from a very full life in California to a simpler one on a small, rural island off the west coast of Canada. I have the privilege to live and work on the unceded territories of the Coast

Salish peoples. My house is in the forest, where the trees speak to me, and the owls and the eagles bless me with their presence. It is my sanctuary home.

Here I work for the Raffi Foundation for Child Honouring, through which, among other things, I bring an ecopsychology and pre- and perinatal lens to the Child Honouring vision. The foundation's mission is to transform society to meet the priority needs of the very young, with "child honouring" proposed as a universal ethic. I also consult with organizations dedicated to indigenous causes and participate in various leadership counsels related to the climate crisis, Breathwork, and of course, Birthing The New Humanity. I am deeply grateful to belong to this wonderful global community of dedicated people.

I still love my therapy practice. It now consists mainly of short-term transformational work with diverse leaders who are committed to creating positive change in the world.

As I look back, it's clear to me that so much of my life has been preparation for this crucible moment.

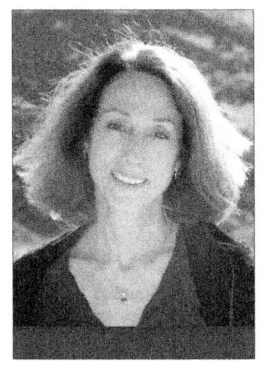

Adela Barcia's focus throughout her professional life has been on creating engaging frameworks for personal and social transformation. She has been a committed peace activist for over 40 years, both on a global level and in the interior worlds of the clients in her psychotherapy practice. Now, viewing the climate emergency as a potential portal for global systemic change, Adela is wholeheartedly dedicating her energy and her skills to this crucible moment.

Chapter 12

A LOVING UNIVERSE

By Dr. Julie Gerland (*hc*)

I laid terrified in my bed, frozen with fear, adrenalin pumping throughout my body. I knew I couldn't fight or run from this situation. *The stranger* was climbing the stairs and was about to enter the room. I heard the handle open the door, and in my mind's eye, I followed the figure, clutching the blanket to my chin, as it moved into the middle of the room.

There was nothing to steal in the room or in any part of the Sussex countryside house our friends had been kind enough to let us stay in. We were a far cry from the hustle and bustle of my native Hong Kong, a city that never sleeps.

Our family was depressed and missing the noise and activities we were all used to. We had come here because my father was out of work, and my parents had used up all their savings. We had no money and were not entitled to any benefits, as they had left the UK when they were young.

"He could take what he wants," I thought. "I'll pretend to be asleep." Far from imagining that my life was about to change forever, I braced for the worse. It was pitch black, and my glare was fixed in the place where I was convinced the strange man stood. Suddenly, the presence turned into a point of Light. I knew this was no ordinary light. It was not unusual for me to see invisible light and color. From my early childhood, I saw things and beings that most people don't. I actually lived in a kind of trance state most of the time.

The point of Light spread throughout the room, moving rapidly towards me. It engulfed me, and instantly, for the first time in my life, I felt completely safe, known, seen, and unconditionally loved. I experienced being an integral part of an immense web of intelligent, loving, and endless life. This was my first taste of mystical bliss, a state that was to become my beloved life companion, my go-to place, my saving grace, my loving universe. It felt like my true inner parents, the ones who see and know me for the Soul I truly am, had come to claim me.

Previously I had often felt unseen, unheard, and unloved, spending hours crying alone in my bed. My physical parents were good people, but like many others, they thought that if their children had food, shelter, and no physical abuse, they were doing a perfect job. However, our goal is to not only survive but also thrive. Our parents' role is to reinforce our true nature and connection with an innately loving and intelligent universe, teaching us to live in harmony with eternal laws.

I promptly fell into a very deep sleep. The next morning, I awoke to my father putting a cup of tea beside my bed. To his surprise, I bolted upright. Previously I had nothing to get up for, no enthusiasm or interest in the day ahead. "There is no point in trying to explain," the calm soft voice said in my head, "he won't be able to understand." Keeping the experience for myself, I went outside where all of nature, every blade of grass, was ablaze with the same Light. The sheep in the neighboring field all came to greet me with a loving gaze. I knew and told my father that he would get a wonderful job, which he soon did. He returned to Hong Kong and left me in England. I was only 16 years old with no money, knowing only a handful of people. Yet, oddly, I felt as old as time, completely safe and supported by Life Itself.

"So why do people suffer?" I asked myself, "Why are we not living as one happy sharing, caring global family?" These questions fueled my burning desire to share this love and bliss with the world. The planet soon became my garden and humanity my family. I had many amazing experiences, including co-creating a children's center in the Hong Kong slums. I met some of the greatest spiritual teachers, activists, and heart-centered people from diverse cultures and traditions, including the great spiritual master Omraam Mikhael Aivanhov.

His phrase, "If we were to look after pregnant women, in just two generations, or fifty years, we could close all our prisons and all our hospitals," gave me the answer to my questions and determined my life's mission.

The time of development in the womb is the missing key to healing ourselves, our families, and the planet. When we deeply understand this process of incarnation, we can transform our limitations, reach our full potential, and thrive.

From the moment of conception, every human being would be aware and consecrated to accomplish their Divine mission, manifesting the splendor of their Soul and Spirit on earth for the highest good of all. They would remember who they truly are and feel safe and free to thrive in a loving, intelligent universe, governed by perfect universal laws.

Diving deep into self-exploration, I loved discovering and experiencing new states of consciousness. Re-visiting and experiencing my own time in the womb and birth allowed me to become aware of how this passage affected me. I also began gathering pregnancy stories and studied how children were subsequently affected.

One of these stories came from my own family. A hot day in Singapore, my mother, pregnant with her first child, screamed when she found a snake in her bedroom. My father immediately came to her rescue and killed the intruder. They later found out that the snake was actually harmless. She was struck by intense remorse that this innocent life had been lost because of her. Ten years later, her son became obsessed with the need to save and nurture snakes. He would buy them from the Chinese market with his pocket money, and some years later he kept Percy the python as his favorite pet. Clearly, his mother's experience and remorse were imprinted on his subconscious mind.

I began teaching children to swim, and soon mothers were bringing me their toddlers. Several were pregnant with their next child. With no formal training, I began helping them deal with the fears, doubts, and stresses they were confronted with. Feeling inadequate and lacking the skills to help them change habits such as smoking, I knew I had to learn how to empower them to change and free themselves from harmful addictions. Challenges and conflict in their relationships were also a major issue, and they confided in me.

The polarity of man and woman has always been a source of deep interest to me. Its understanding is clearly a missing key to creating a harmonious family life. At first, I learnt from observing my parents who separately talked to me about their feelings of frustration and emotional pain. Engaged to be married at the tender age of 15, my own relationships started early. I discovered that sexual passion often provoked misunderstandings, possessiveness, and jealousy. Even tender and real love didn't seem to have the power to overcome this source of separation and hurt. The possibility of living a spiritual marriage, where we could blossom together on every level of our being, eluded me. At the age of 21, I decided that I would live a celibate life.

Five years later, François and I became close spiritual friends. One day we experienced something that neither of us had ever dreamt possible. Just after a meditation, a powerful yet subtle union of pure love and light took place as we sat opposite each other, across a table. Our energies suddenly merged, and we felt as if we were one. From that moment on, the deep secrets of polarity began to unveil themselves before us.

In 1989, we bought an old farmhouse in the foothills of the French Pyrenees. It soon became a center for early parenting, spiritual retreats, and intense inner work. One day, the American psychologist, hypnotherapist, and author Dr. David Chamberlain and his wife Donna came to stay with us. They are two of the most beautiful human beings I have met. David, one of the fathers of contemporary prenatal psychology, was compiling scientific evidence from medical journals about prenatal development and newborn babies. The discoveries were startling.

A group of passionate professionals gathered here at Providence to hear him. He said he had great success simply "asking babies to turn" into the vertex position when their mothers, allergic to anesthesia, were threatened with a cesarean section. He showed us that prenatal and newborn babies are conscious, intelligent, and participating in their experience of birth. Life is intelligent, and when we learn how to communicate with love and respect, it becomes so much simpler.

My holistic parenting program was already attracting some early European adopters. During his visit, David encouraged me to include natural birth classes. I knew nothing about birth and needed to learn about a process that I was not ready to experience. François and I never felt that our mission in life was to have children. I had been taught and wrongly believed that birth was a medical event.

When I heard about the pioneer of HypnoBirthing, Marie Mongan, I knew I had found what I needed. I flew to the USA to train in her childbirth education method. Delighted, I began teaching couples this new extension of my work, and a few years later I became a faculty member to train professionals.

The Mongan Method is taught in over 47 countries and has revolutionized the way mums and dads birth their babies.

Thanks to HypnoBirthing, many couples now experience birth as a joyful, naturally comfortable celebration of life. They are no longer afraid of a natural physiological process designed by an incredible, loving intelligence. They are taking birth back from a dominating, fear-driven, and over-medicalized system. The birth process is being reborn into the power of intimacy and a loving, evolved nest. I still enjoy busting the all-too-prevalent myths, including that birth is meant to be painful. It is not! However, the condition for this is the absence of fear and stress and the presence of oxytocin, the love hormone. Yes, giving birth is designed to be an act of love when we cast off the shadows of fear and separation and, like the prodigal child, return home to our Loving Universe.

I didn't have the privilege of being born under such conditions. I discovered later how much my birth had affected me. For years I couldn't stand being hurried to leave my room, being told I was late or holding someone up. I would have strong emotional reactions, finding myself taking even longer to get ready. This, I discovered, was triggering my birth trauma.

The subconscious memory of being violently induced at birth by my mother, under medical supervision, was still vivid inside me. She had taken castor oil to artificially start the birth, even though there was no medical emergency. This was the deep cause of my discomfort and behavior.

Most people are unaware of the lifelong consequences of obstetrical interventions often performed for convenience or financial reasons or to justify the use of expensive equipment. Mothers and their partners are being sold the high-risk fear mongering and dramatization which is often the very cause of complications. They are not being warned of the long-term psychological and physical consequences of this obstetric violence.

It is nevertheless possible to change our buried memories and stop passing on intergenerational limitations, violence, and suffering. When future parents do this work before conceiving, they will have a more positive pregnancy, creating deep and lasting bonds of love with their baby and enjoying a better birth experience. Our BirthTheChange® curriculum is designed to empower people to heal trauma, change subconscious programs, and access their immense reservoir of inner possibilities. Everyone can change the past and create the future of their dreams. As we often say, "It is never too late to have a happy childhood."

Unfortunately, becoming aware of this new paradigm, some parents experience shame or guilt that they haven't done the right thing with their previous children. I tell them they did the best they could with what they knew – that's all they could do. That's all we'll ever do. A child doesn't feel guilty because he fell over when learning to walk. In the same way, we also continue to develop and naturally improve. Let's accept what we have done with the best intentions and choose to embrace continual learning and developing as a way of life.

Bringing a new being to the planet is a sacred and life-changing process. It takes preparation, knowledge, and inner work to be a good role model and pass on the best qualities. It is possible to lay the foundations for the incoming Soul to thrive in a human body and thus regenerate humanity.

Nothing is more important than the birthing process. It guides me in all I do and applies to everything we wish to create. Mother Nature has given us the perfect process for us to birth our most lofty ideas into matter. Consciously preparing, conceiving, developing, birthing, and nurturing has become our way of life. We have created the Conscious Creation Plan® to empower people to live in harmony with nature, succeed in their endeavors, and participate in "bringing heaven on earth." We all have the power to create, and our destiny is to become conscious creators.

The Great Mother is calling us to awaken. Wiping away our tears and sorrows, She is birthing the new humanity. We can choose to rejoice as we go through the passage ending an era of fear, struggle, and survival. We are being born into the Light of a Loving Universe where we are safe, loved, connected, and guided by Her intelligence. We are witnessing the dawn of a new era where thriving starts in the womb and lasts a lifetime.

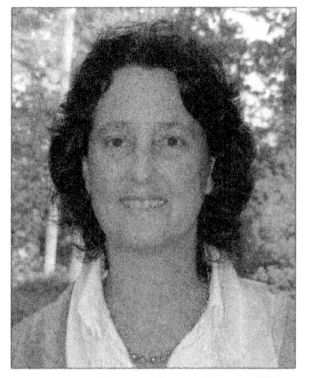 **Dr. Julie Gerland (*hc*)** has been a pioneer and thought leader for over forty years, dedicated to achieving a thriving global family and planet. She was awarded an honorary doctorate in Holistic Medicines, and she is the co-founder of Birthing The New Humanity, BTNH World, BirthTheChange®, and the Conscious Creation Plan®. She is an inspiring international speaker, TEDx presenter, best-selling co-author, HypnoBirthing Trainer, and a social entrepreneur.

To connect: https://birthingthenewhumanity.com + download the Birthing The New Humanity App.

Chapter 13

HEALING SPACE

By Marilyn Mitchell, MD

We all start our existence with two cells merging, and then a whole human being is formed in just nine months with all systems on go. This is "scientifically impossible" to describe or to reproduce in a lab. When those two cells merge, the energy field (the lifeforce) surrounds them, and that provides the information that informs those two little cells to grow into a human being. This is the process that selects which genes to turn on and turn off and gives the instruction for the human body to form.

The energy that surrounds us at conception, and those energy fields that form, stay with us through our entire lives. They have been measured, the largest one being our heart energy. It can be measured about 10 feet spherically around the body, and it dominates the other energies. These fields start forming at conception and through pregnancy, and then commit to the body and stay with it at the time of birth.

How do I know this? It was revealed to me through the course of my life...

As a child, I listened to an intuitive part of myself, and this information seemed precious and private. I also loved school and loved informational and linear learning. As I went through my life, I began to have experiences in which my intuitive nature would start to blend into my work.

When I was in college, I received guidance that I should go to medical school, which totally surprised me, because I thought, "The doctors aren't very much about health." But I followed that guidance and learned medicine, and at the same time I learned about energy healing. I was learning how to access energy, and an intuitive healing power.

When I was a medical student I was allowed to deliver a baby. It was such a profound experience that I thought, *I want to be in this space all the time.* That led me into women's health, and an OB/GYN residency. It was in that moment of birthing, while delivering a baby, that I recognized the powerful lifeforce and energy shifts that occur in the body.

And then I had another teaching. I became curious about our body's energies when I was pregnant for the first time. I had a question that I put out to the universe: "When does the soul actually commit to the body, to stay there? When does that energy commit?" I waited for an answer, and when I was in labor and it was getting very intense, I popped out of my body and was watching from above.

At a certain point, the nurse said, "It's time to push." I thought, "Oh, I don't want to go back in my body." I was reluctant. Next, I saw a light over in the distance that was coming, coming, coming down towards my body below. Then I observed that it went in and actually entered my daughter's body, and right after that I returned – Whoosh! – into my body, and realized we both were birthed at the same time. I was taught that the lifeforce commits to the life at birth. I realized also that I was being birthed into motherhood as she was being birthed into this lifetime.

I had that experience whenever I delivered a baby after that. The energy is with the embryo, but that freedom commits to the body at birth. It stays then with the body.

I realized my real mission was to introduce people to that huge energy resource that we have but are not taught to access.

We founded a very large women's health practice in OB/GYN. After some time, I had an experience that was quite powerful where I saw inside the body before starting an emergency surgery, and I knew exactly what to do to save the woman's life. That's when I realized it was important that I bring those skills to people. I completed formal training in Energy Healing, and we brought Energy Healing into the practice.

Today, after serving as an obstetrician for 25 years, I founded a practice called HealingSpace where we see both men and women. We do energy healing and some traditional and integrative medicine, and we get people's physical bodies working without medicines. We get thyroids working. We've had some profound cancer reversal. We teach people how to access their healing energy for themselves. One of the biggest blocks is mental. We have been taught to try to solve everything from our mind, but we have a greater source of healing power that is innate.

Most people come in because something's going on physically, and they're not able to get to the bottom of it. Medicine is not really answering their concerns. Much of the time I'm sitting with someone and realizing that there's some block or something that's happened that is preventing them from bringing their full life force to the situation

I introduce people to their lifeforce ability. This force is our birthright. We receive it at birth and we have access to it our whole lives, but no one teaches us how to use it. At HealingSpace we teach our patients how to access it for themselves, and then we also do energy work during sessions with them so that the healing can be supported more. A number of people come to me who are starting their families. Although I'm not delivering babies anymore, I do help them through the process and introduce them to the connection they seek as they start their families.

We are bombarded with media and social pressure, we have learned that we must try to figure out our lives, to do everything in our heads. It's a relief to many people to experience that connection to their vital life force. There are some very simple ways to retrain our minds and get back to using our intuitive healing force. Women that come during menopause, for example, upon introducing them to that part of them that's always able to heal, I help them shift their focus, and they can bring that then to their spouses, children and others.

The healing force actually kicks in even when we take a medicine. It's that healing part of us, that energetic part of us that does the healing with the nudge of some medicine. Anytime we have an ailment, that energy has been blocked. We're not getting enough of the energy that makes us thrive.

I teach people some easy techniques in which they can get their mind to quiet and listen to and cultivate that deeper intuitive part. Instead of Googling and worrying and just narrating their life all the time, I teach them to get their mind to be the implementer and to listen to the intuitive. If someone is sick, it's particularly important to help them basically get their mind redirected toward healing.

Often, our minds keep reiterating how bad we feel or what's wrong. They have to figure it out. That actually makes things worse. My practice implements techniques to quiet the mind and get it to listen for instruction from that intuitive, energetic, soulful part of us. I introduce people to that huge resource that they have and can retrain their mind to its rightful importance. So instead of unwittingly making things worse, it's actually listening for direction so that it can understand the real source of what's going on and help to be part of the solution rather than grinding in the problem.

Fear originates in the mind, and fear can make you sick. It can inhibit that natural lifeforce that we have in our immune system for one thing. That's one of the trickiest things about this pandemic: people have felt very fearful and disempowered that it can weaken the body. We have been able to bring people back to that trust in their own body and help them stay out of fear.

The first thing is to recognize that our minds can be runaway. Of course, meditation is great if people can do that. There's a wonderful, very simple technique that you can apply if you have racy mind, and you just need it to stop: Relax your tongue and the voice can't speak. It's powerful. I teach that to people in the office, and it's huge. It's a great way to help people who have trouble sleeping, falling asleep, or staying asleep. What I added was that you relax the tongue and the mind quiets and is present and still, but it's not talking. Then you can retrain that part of your mind that really wants to serve. We give it a job that actually helps. For sleep, you put it in charge of guarding the sleep, and then you relax the tongue and go to sleep. If you wake up, you catch it before it goes, "Oh no, I'm awake." That's a simple technique.

Other times we can relax the tongue and ask for our minds to listen to the intuitive part of the brain. So, if you're facing an illness for example, get quiet, relax the tongue, and ask the mind to listen to what's going on, rather than worrying about it.

Another technique is just to get into that quiet space, pose the question that you have about yourself, and then let it go. For me, the answer usually pops up in the shower the next morning. In this way, we can reorganize how the mind and the soulful, intuitive, energetic part can work together in a more positive, healthful way.

Especially in Western culture, people become depressed, having no idea how much more alive they could be. Through birthing into humanity, people can understand that they can possess that incredible lifeforce that we have when we're coming in being born throughout their lives. People can even choose their time to leave this earth. We know about cultures that do that. We can shift our lives and have healthier and happier and more fulfilling lives by just realizing we have that access.

Many native cultures access this and use it very regularly. By bringing it more to Western cultures, through knowledge among physicians and other providers, we could definitely shift our health and even our inspiration and our enjoyment of life.

Fear limits our ability to really thrive during this lifetime, and just introducing people to that other source could make an enormous difference in how we treat one another and how we treat the earth that we depend on. There would be much less fear and more collaboration. It would be really nice, for example, to make pharma unnecessary or less necessary. People could be healthier and more cooperative. Having more people live from that place could change businesses and systems so that we're living in a more communal, cooperative world.

Western cultures have gone off the deep end in terms of mind and accumulation and moved away from spirit. It might be that we have more of a blending of the native way of thinking with our Western orientation. I think it could make a wonderful transformation.

My purpose in coming into this life was to bring this awareness to people. It's certainly my joy to do that. It has felt like the most wonderful knowledge that's unfolded to me, and I've been able to help others with it in a very profound way. I feel very blessed to have the life that I am experiencing.

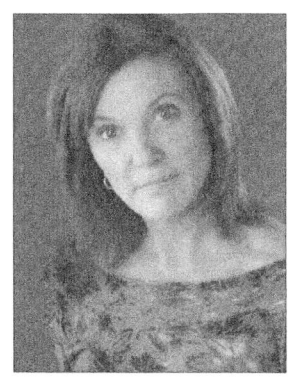

Marilyn Mitchell, M.D., has spent 40 years cultivating a unique practice that integrates Energy Healing with holistic and traditional medicine: HealingSpace Medical Center, St. Charles, Illinois. She earned her M.D. from Rush Medical College, Board Certifications in Obstetrics/Gynecology and Integrative/Holistic Medicine and certifications by Barbara Brennan School of Healing and EnergyTouch School of Advanced Healing. She is author of *The True Nature of Healing: A Surgeon's Soul Journey* and the *WiseWoman Menopause Workbook* at www.healingspacellc.com.

See also www.reimagininghealthcare.org.

Chapter 14

A MEDICINE FOR OUR TIME

Harnessing the power of Music to Welcome Healthy Babies into Our World

By Gary Malkin

For thousands of years, the world's spiritual visionaries have believed that the rational mind alone will never be able to solve our most intractable challenges. Many can argue that most of the world's problems are exacerbated by an over-reliance on reductionist science and hyper-rationalism. But a global movement of forward-thinking visionaries steeped in quantum science believes that our dominating linear minds must now be tempered and experienced through a more potent force: the wisdom of the human heart.

What modality might have the capacity to awaken the heart's wisdom most effectively?

Of all the existing art forms, the one that can efficiently impact our biochemistry, activate our neurotransmitters, stimulate oxytocin-induced compassion, and reduce stress is one that can shift our vibrational field at the cellular level: The immersive listening phenomenon known as *music*.

The language of music is universal. It speaks to each human heart in its own dialect, in ways that touch and ignite precisely what is needed for that heart to open and bloom. Music holds a key that unlocks the human soul, long held in myopic confinement by the logical eloquence and dominance of our rational minds. Music utilizes our senses to go "under the radar" by directly reaching our subconscious minds – the area from which most of our behavior, identity, and sense of meaning originates.

From time immemorial, music has been shaping our ceremonies, rituals, and gatherings with sounds that were designed to inspire, unify, soothe, heal, and awaken us to a recognition of the miracle of life itself. The vibration of string, the whisper of wind, the rhythmic pulse of skin and wood, along with the intimacy of the human voice – such sounds can take us to expanded vistas within ourselves, liberating us into the full range of human emotions.

When we deeply listen to heart-opening music, we experience greater presence, inner peace, gratitude, and a sense of belonging that feels like *home*. Then we feel more comfortable to share feelings that are more often left unexpressed, revealing new perspectives on our lives. This shared intimacy strengthens bonds with our loved ones during these meaningful transitions of our lives. Then our disarmed defenses organically evolve into a blessed recognition of that which matters most. Mystics refer to this experience as 'Grace', a transpersonal state that has been restoring human beings to the best versions of themselves since the beginning of time.

Sadly, 'civilized' cultures have long believed that these expressions of emotional vulnerability would best be subjugated due to the cultural pressure to be seen as credible by predominantly communicating with an over-reliance on the linear, rational mind. But during our shared life transitions, the right music can crack us open, revealing tender, sensitive feelings. This vulnerability has been affirmed by the acclaimed social researcher *Brene Brown*, who shares that these genuine feelings are the source of our authenticity, our uniqueness and an innocence that is at the very core of our humanity.

All this brings us to what this chapter is all about: how life-generative music and sound can provide peaceful strategies for parents who want to provide the most optimal care for their babies at all stages of development. As we increasingly understand the damaging impact of stress - especially on those who are bringing new life into our harsh world - it's essential that we provide accessible forms of respite from the chaotic conditions of contemporary life during these challenging times. Whether through extemporaneous lullabies, guided meditations, or music for our environments, music can offer a *balm* for the heart and soul that can shift parents from being stressed, impatient, and emotionally reactive to being resilient, self-aware, and grateful for the miracle of having a new baby.

One can only imagine how stressful birthing and rearing new life into the world can be. Most of us are coming and going at an alarming pace, even without children. It has become the norm for new parents to rush through their many obligations, engaging with their ever-absorbing digital devices while multitasking with baby in arms, compromising everyone's sense of well-being in more ways than they ever thought possible.

Rather than repeatedly subjecting our babies to adrenaline-rich *fight-flight-freeze* behaviors that can negatively impact their delicate nervous systems, calming musical strategies can contribute to the formation of a baby's healthy psychological foundation while supporting the *birthing of a new humanity* based on humane values, wellness, and emotional coherence.

The cultural epidemic of doing too much and moving too quickly continues to adversely affect us all. This is especially true for those struggling to survive in developing cultures, where basic needs might not consistently be met, creating dangerous levels of survival stress. But no matter what the circumstances, it's vital to protect all parents' capacities so that our babies could evolve into physiologically and emotionally healthy human beings. Intentionally listening to life-generative music can make a meaningful difference in the well-being for all concerned.

It is well known that the parents need to deeply connect with their baby in a multitude of ways. As important as mother's milk, babies need to feel their parent's loving presence as they bond during the first hours, days, and months of life. New studies show that this attachment capacity is even true for babies developing inside the womb - and music can support this bonding process while mitigating life's stresses with nourishing states of heart coherence, gratitude, and awe.

Birthing The New Humanity cofounder, Julie Gerland states:

"Sound is like welding. It goes straight into and becomes part of matter. Sound contributes to the symmetry and constitution of our bodies, because we know that matter can be affected and formed by sound."

Did you know that the first sense to arrive at 24 weeks in utero, is our hearing sense? And did you know that everything in the universe - from the smallest subatomic particles to the greatest spheres in the cosmos - is made up of vibrations? When we engage in the vibrational language of music during this seminal stage of life, we are directly impacting our lives on a vibrational level where the frequencies in our bodies' molecules will catalyze biochemical reactions that will either promote health and wellness or negative conditions that could last a lifetime.

As for me, I dreamed of being a film composer at an early age, and ultimately received professional training at schools such as USC and Oberlin Conservatory. During the first twenty years of my professional career, I created original music for hundreds of television, film, and commercial projects while I cultivated the ability to musically elicit deep emotional responses from audiences.

I was approached by my dear friend and musical visionary Michael Stillwater. He and his wife Doris invited me to musically explore how we might be able to support people to find acceptance of the dying process, especially after all attempts to heal were exhausted. We recorded many heart-opening spoken messages from well-known visionaries such as dying pioneer, *Elisabeth Kubler Ross*, spiritual teacher, *Ram Das*, the Buddhist teacher, *Thich Nath Hanh*, and the esteemed *Rabbi Zalman Shacter-Shelomi*. I applied the aesthetics of film scoring to these tender spoken messages, enhancing them with a poignant orchestral score.

Since *Graceful Passages: A Companion for Living and Dying* was released, it has helped hundreds of thousands of people to reconsider the dying process - not as something to fear - but as a meaningful spiritual experience that could be accepted as part of the natural cycle of life. During this time, I learned how powerfully music could be utilized to navigate and assimilate loss. I came to discover that my life's purpose was to harness my musical talents to serve others by illuminating, inspiring, and supporting those going through the significant passages of life.

A few years after *Graceful Passages* received global acclaim, I met sound healer and spiritual guide *Lisa Rafel*. As a new grandmother, Lisa had started creating soulful lullabies designed for new parents so they could slow down and use these songs to connect more with the miracle of new life.

Against the backdrop of pregnancy and birth being increasingly over-medicalized in mainstream healthcare, she and her husband, clinical psychologist *David Surrenda, Ph.D.* invited me to co-create musical ways to welcome new life into the world. We became fascinated with how these songs might strengthen the attachment bonding process for parents and newborns and started collaborating towards these objectives.

As we did this, the science of epigenetics empowered us to create musical resources that could inspire healthy, empowered choices so that parents and babies would have a strong emotional connection from the beginning. Epigenetics teaches us that it is not just our genes that affect our life script, but the ways intention and energy are added to the process that potentiate genes being activated (or not). Given this new understanding, the ramifications of music's impact on this tender phase of life cannot be overestimated.

Our first project, *Safe in the Arms of Love: Deepening the Essential Bond with Your Baby* demonstrates how powerfully a coherent emotional state of the parent can positively impact their baby's well-being. This award-winning gift-book combines beautiful, intentionally designed music, parent-directed lyrics, and easy-to-understand information about the importance of securing a strong emotional foundation for a child's entire life. We then created a collection of evocative songs to strengthen a mother's capacity for prenatal bonding called *"The Journey of Our Lives"*.

Our evidence-based hospital studies have clinically shown that when a mother listens to our music while holding her baby (who is not hearing the music), the mother is calmed into heartfelt coherence, positively impacting her baby's vitals of oxygen saturation and heart rate variability. These states corresponded to positive biochemical responses such as more oxytocin, healthy vagus nerve activity, and serotonin production, all supporting the inherent ability to love, connect, and self-regulate.

An excerpt from a chapter written by Lisa in *Safe in the Arms of Love* sheds further light:

"Even in the womb, your baby is listening to you. When beautiful music enters this little world, vibrations caress the multiplying cells that are becoming your baby. The rocking vibrations are gently absorbed like an elixir into the tiny nervous

system. Loving words are like music as well. The tone is important. The vibration of your voice establishes the connection for how your baby knows you when it is born. Your baby enters this world with eyes that cannot see. Through your voice, your baby recognizes who you are.

Once your baby is born, everything that happens around the baby takes on great significance. Some cultures believe the transition from the womb to the world needs special care. When the baby lies skin to skin on its parent's chest, heart on heart, the physical health and attachment of both mother and baby is supported.

Often songs are sung to establish the bond even more. Music stimulates development in the brain at multiple levels and the newborn's brain has one billion neurons. Each neuron forms up to 15,000 separate connections, leading to more than 50 trillion synapses, forming more connections than all the stars in the universe!

By utilizing the psychoacoustics of rhythm, tempo, pitch, and intention (what we refer to as Positive Intention Music™), the songs and music of Safe in the Arms of Love support an atmosphere in which both parent and baby can be emotionally connected."

Dr. David Surrenda, whose deep knowledge of the parent-child relationship informs all the work we've been creating, says:

"Bonding is one of the most important steps in a child's development, helping to build strong and meaningful relationships in the future. Through the coherent qualities of gentle, loving music, we wanted to create clear reference points for parents to learn this natural and universal experience."

Our latest collaboration, a social-impact theatrical musical play entitled *"Can You Hear Me Baby?* harnesses the power of heartwarming and poignant theatrical storytelling and songs to inspire individuals from all walks of life to bring new beings into the world with greater ease, health, and awareness for all involved. Our dream is to birth this thought-provoking musical into mainstream culture soon, and we look forward to receiving support from the global conscious birthing community when it is launched into the world.

With all that we understand about these sensitive beings growing inside and outside the womb, utilizing music to generate a consistent experience of "all is well" promotes a more conscious stewardship of this precious passage in life, ultimately helping us as a society to strengthen the cellular foundation from which our incoming generations can be born into a world where everyone can thrive.

Through the transformative power of music, we hope to support the growing movement of social artists, healers, and visionaries who are utilizing their creative gifts to create a world where incoming generations will be given unconditional love and respect, imbuing them with a reverence for the sacredness of all life.

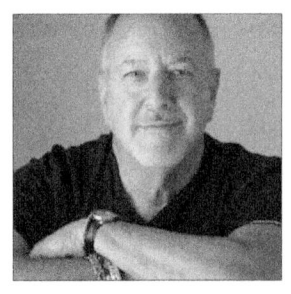 **Gary Malkin** is a multiple Emmy award-winning composer, performer, and public speaker whose career in film, television, and commercial music spans more than thirty years. For the last twenty years, his groundbreaking work has been re-defining music's role as a resource for healing and activating flow states. His globally acclaimed listening resource, Graceful Passages, co-created with Michael and Doris Stillwater, has provided support for people to face life's losses with greater compassion and acceptance. Frequently keynoting on global webinars, Gary produces humanizing musical interventions that address many of the challenges facing our society today. He is a member of the Association for Transformational Leaders and the

Evolutionary Leaders Circle. You can experience his music at
WisdomoftheWorld.com.

Chapter 15

THE MESSAGE OF WATER

By Michiko Hayashi

I had just started a three-month vacation in March 2004 when I bought books on Hado ("vibration" in Japanese) that were to determine my life's mission. Two of the books were written by Masaru Emoto; one was about Hado, and the other was about water and its relation to vibration. I was astonished by the deep content and learnt the most important law of the universe from them. My father became a Buddhist priest when I was young and showed me how to appreciate, respect, and be kind to everyone and everything around me. The water crystals that I saw in Dr. Emoto's books revealed to me that what my father taught me was right. Love and gratitude are very beautiful vibrations. This IS the truth. It was my fate to work with Dr. Emoto, and I am very grateful that the universe gave me this precious opportunity.

Before Dr. Emoto started to conduct research on water, he was a doctor of alternative medicine for over 10 years and had helped more than 10,000 people with his Hado device and Water. Back then, he was very well known as the pioneer and master of Hado in Japan. When I read his book on Hado, I was amazed at the profound knowledge he had and shared. In that book, I learned that everything was vibration, and from a vibrational point of view, everything has positive and negative sides, including our emotions, and that the same vibrations are attracted to each other through the phenomena of resonance.

For example, irritation has the same Hado (vibration) as mercury (Hg). So, when we are irritated, we are emanating the same vibration as mercury, thus mercury resonates with us in the perspective of Hado. Sadness has the same vibration as aluminum, so if I am in deep sadness, I am attracting aluminum. The balance of vibration is very important. There is Yin and Yang, but there is a middle as well. The best is to be well balanced, not too positive and not too negative. Each part of our organs has its intrinsic Hado, and when it exists out of the intrinsic vibration for some time, then we begin to have problems in that very part of our physical body.

However, there is no need to worry, because as mentioned above, everything has yin and yang, negative and positive just like darkness and light. So, by changing the negative emotion to positive, we can neutralize the vibration, and thus we create harmony within. From the Hado perspective, the negative side of appreciation is resentment. When you notice that you are holding a grudge, you can neutralize such negative Hado by changing it to gratitude. To do that, you may want to see something you love so you feel grateful, or you can simply say "thank you" many times to whatever you appreciate.

We can always neutralize the vibration of our negative or positive emotions. In the case of someone feeling lonely or sad for a long time, he or she attracts aluminum. Aluminum is one of the big causes of Alzheimer's. So when we feel lonely or sad, we can do something fun to cheer ourselves up. As such, we will stop attracting aluminum. As Hado is the foundation of everything and all phenomena, learning about Hado helps us improve our health and life as well as our environment, including Mother Earth, which is the beautiful and precious home of all living beings.

Here are some of the emotions that share the same Hado of positive and negative.

Negative emotion : Positive emotion

Resentment ⇔ Appreciation

Anger ⇔ Kindness

Fear ⇔ Courage

Anxiety ⇔ Security

Irritation ⇔ Poise

Pressure ⇔ Calmness

As Dr. Emoto had the profound knowledge of Hado, he treated so many people with his Hado device and water. He knew that water has memory and delivers information. This is how he went into the research on water.

The other book of Dr. Emoto's that I read was about water and included many photos of ice water crystals. I did not know of this concept or had seen such pictures before. When I saw the water crystals after being exposed to "Thank you", "You fool" and "Love and Gratitude", I had goosebumps, and I instantaneously knew it was the truth of nature. Dr. Emoto said that water absorbs the frequency of each word, and water crystals are the visualization of Hado. I was fascinated by his research and Hado. I visited his website only to discover he needed someone to help him with the copyright of his books. This was the beginning of my journey with Dr. Emoto in 2004.

He announced at the United Nations Headquarters in May 2005 that he would be writing a children's book from *The Message from Water* and give 650 million children's books to children for free so that they can learn to live in harmony within themselves and with others. It became his most important work. He also founded the non-profit organization The Emoto Peace Project to share the important truth of water. This was to become known as the discovery of Masaru Emoto. You probably know that the human body is made up of approximately 70% water.

Mother Earth is also about 70% water. We are all born in water. Without water, nothing can stay alive. Water IS life.

What if every water molecule has memory? Are we giving beautiful information to water in our body and around us? We are breathing in water in the air. Our skin is absorbing water in the air. What if water is deeply connected to our consciousness? Our mind is busy thinking about many things and constantly having emotions. Study says that the average person has 30,000–60,000 thoughts per day. As our thoughts and emotions are vibration, and vibration is energy, we are constantly emitting energy and creating an invisible field with our consciousness.

Our thoughts and emotions become words, and then they become actions. Our thoughts, emotions, words, and actions affect our health, life, family, society, and this precious earth, because they are all Hado (vibration). It is now accepted in mainstream science that water has memory, and water is the conductor of our consciousness. Let me explain this idea.

Masaru Emoto conducted extensive water research, and through more than tens of thousands of frozen water crystal photos taken at his laboratory, he discovered that, when water is exposed to positive, beautiful words, thoughts, and music, water creates beautiful hexagonal crystalline structures, as water absorbs the vibration of such beautiful thoughts, words, and everything around it. On the other hand, when water is exposed to something negative, ugly, or destructive, it doesn't make crystalline structures but rather forms ugly or misshapen forms.

Water responds to all vibrations at the molecular level. The most beautiful and brilliant crystal that water made comes after exposure to two words together: *love* and *gratitude*. By learning from water, and because both humans and the planet earth are almost water, we all shall be loving, grateful, respectful, kind, and honest and shall act accordingly instead of being negative, angry, worried, critical, and destructive. By living positively and kindly with love and gratitude, we become physically well and happy, and our lives become positive and beautiful.

This discovery also shows that we humans are creating our reality almost with just our thoughts and words. When we think, and thoughts are vibrations and energy, the same vibration resonates. Therefore, the same vibration will come back to you as a phenomenon of the same vibration. For example, when you throw a stone into the water in a pond, it makes waves (vibration), and ultimately the waves return to where the stone was thrown. When you are happy, you are emitting a happy vibration, and so something that makes you happy will return to you as a result. This is the law of Hado vibration; it is the law of the Universe and the law of attraction.

Babies grow in the amniotic liquid in their mother's womb. They have the memory from the time of conception or even before that. It is very beneficial for everyone to know this. Babies in the womb are feeling what their mothers are feeling, because water carries the vibration. If a mother is happy, her baby is happy. This has a big impact on the baby's whole life. If the mother is listening to something beautiful, the baby is feeling very calm and peaceful because of the beautiful vibration that the amniotic water is absorbing. This is why it is so very important for all mothers to be in a good and happy state of emotions when they are pregnant. What a big responsibility all mothers have, don't they!? And it is not only the mother's responsibility, but it is the fathers' as well. To help mothers be happy, it is very important that their husbands understand this law of vibration and water. We all want our children to grow to be happy and healthy individuals. How can we raise all of our children happy and healthy? It is quite simple! We must raise them with love and gratitude. We discovered that ignoring a baby in the womb is even worse than having negative words or thoughts.

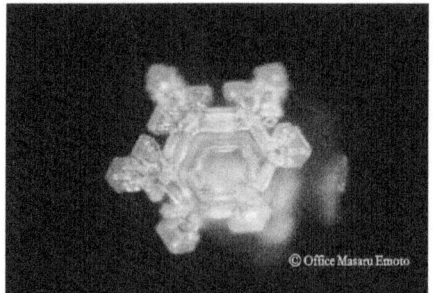

Water crystal of amniotic fluid (diluted 50,000 times).

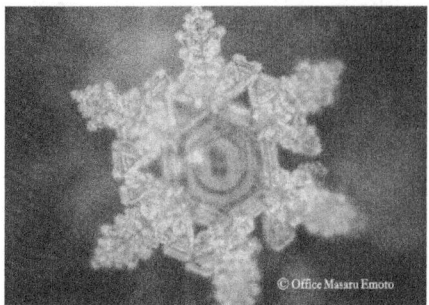

Amniotic fluid after showing the words, "I love you".

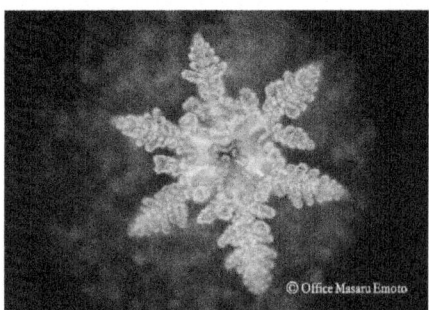

Amniotic fluid exposed to the picture of a smiling girl.

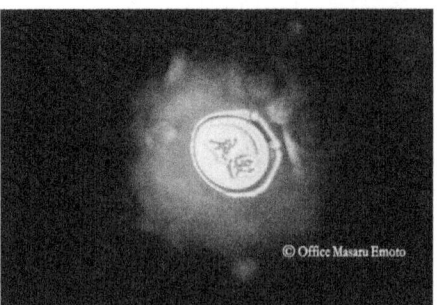

Amniotic fluid exposed to the word "abortion".

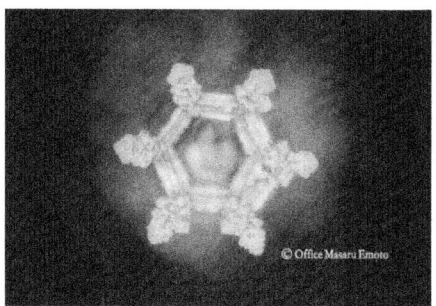

Amniotic fluid exposed to the music "The Four Seasons" by Vivaldi.

If children learn to live positively and kindly from the moment of conception, receiving lots of love, respect, and attention from their parents, they will grow to be loving, kind, respectful, and self-confident. Then their life will be in harmony within, with all around them, and with nature, and thus they will have a happy life. We all have choices every second; do we want to choose to smile at others, or do we want to choose to be grumpy? Do we want to say "thank you," or do we want to take kind actions for granted? Do we want to be kind, or do we want to be mean? Every choice we make creates an invisible field of energy, and it will become a collective energy as a whole. The more loving and kind people there are on earth, the happier people will be and thus the better the world will become.

Here I would like to mention babies, animals, insects, plants, trees, and all beings. They may not look like they understand our languages and circumstances, but they do feel the vibration of what is happening and how people treat them. All living beings have their own ways of communication, and they are very different from that of humans, but that does not mean that they don't have consciousness. They do, just like we do. Babies have not learned how to express their feelings with words yet, but they feel every vibration around them. It is so important that we adults talk to them lovingly and give them respect and much attention with love and gratitude, so they will grow to reach their full potential and thrive.

Almost everyone has a smartphone today, so parents are often so busy looking at their phone even though their babies or children need their attention. Parents don't mean to ignore their children, or they might not even be aware that this action of being busy with phones and paying less attention to their own children is like ignoring their children. Just imagine, when these children are grownups after being raised in this manner, will they know how to love themselves? Will they know how to be kind to others? Will they have self-confidence? Will they have a healthy and happy life? Parents' responsibility is simple: to love their children unconditionally. Children are growing every second, and this process will not wait for you to stop paying attention to something else, such as your phone. This is why it's so important to pay attention to your children with unconditional love whenever they want you. Phones and other things can wait for you to find the time later.

I strongly recommend that you do experiments with something like rice, fruits, seeds, plants, water, or anything alive around you as you see the photos of the "Rice Experiment". When you do your own experiment, you can really tell how powerful the words you are using daily are. Our consciousness and words can create a beautiful life, good health, and improve our environment by choosing to think positive thoughts and by being kind. This is how we all want to live. The world population is now more than 7 billion, and these 7 billion people are energy. It is my hope that every 7 billion people are born and raised with much love, gratitude, and respect, so all 7 billion people will be living harmoniously and peacefully. Needless to say, this whole world will become a beautiful, peaceful, and harmonious place. We are one small part of this planet earth. Every single person, every single being matters.

As I succeeded the late Masaru Emoto's life's mission, Emoto Peace Project, I deliver the Message from Water around the world so that everyone will benefit from it and so that the planet earth will be a healthy, harmonious, and peaceful place.

The invisible field of consciousness is related to our immunity, the well-being of all people, all living beings around us, and ultimately this Mother Earth. Everyone is creating their own life with their consciousness, and as a whole it becomes the collective unconscious mind of this earth.

Emoto left his physical body in 2014, and since then I have been sharing the Message from Water with everyone around the world as well as continuing to do research on water with my team in our Institute. Water crystal photos are the visualization of vibration.

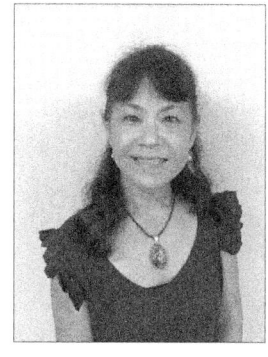 **Michiko Hayashi** is the Global Director and Ambassador of The Emoto Peace Project. She was a personal assistant to Masaru Emoto, the founder and pioneer of Hado ("vibration"), researcher, and best-selling author of *The Message from Water*. Michiko is the successor of his legacy and an international speaker spreading the message of water.

www.EmotoPeaceProject.net

Chapter 16

A WEED IN THE RIVER

By Nutan L Pandit

The common thread in my life has been of abandonment, of rejection, and of not feeling good enough. It probably came from the womb. I was my mother's seventh pregnancy. Preceding me were four sisters, a brother, and a deceased sister. How tired my mother must have been. She must have prayed I would be a boy. In the womb, I must have sensed her yearning, and, being a girl, already felt rejection before being born. That is probably why this has been a dominant emotion in my life.

After a generous dose of Hindi movies in which mothers are extolled as virtuous, never in the wrong, always wishing well for their children, I felt there was something quite not right with me. As an adult, I now realise that our parents are as human as any other human being. That it is possible for a mother, or for that matter, a father, not to love a child.

As I grew up, I had a very large nose and surmised that one of the reasons I was so unlikeable was my big nose. I became painfully conscious of it. Those days we used to see movies in movie halls, and if we arrived late and crossed the beam of light from the projector when navigating towards our seats, people were agitated because it blocked their view. I felt that when I crossed the beam they were more agitated than usual because of my nose! I was painfully conscious of my profile. To make things worse, comic books always showed pirates with my kind of nose!

Finally, I had plastic surgery done on my nose. As luck would have it, a friend of mine suggested I wear an artificial nose ring a few days after my surgery. It turned out that it was too early after my surgery to wear it, and it made my nose crooked again! But I was quite happy because the hump on my nose was gone. The doctor said we could do another surgery to correct it, but I declined.

When I grew up, I went for psycho-therapist counselling over the years but was not helped. I also went to healers, and fortunately, that was useful. One healer asked me to imagine me and my mother together in a garden and then to imagine that we look at each other in the eye and have a conversation. I had great difficulty with it. Then it occurred to me that, in all my 37 years on this planet, my mother had never looked at me in the eye! Until then I had not realised this fact.

As a child, I remember going through traumatic dental treatment. In those days, the dental drill and other equipment were very primitive. Orthodontic dentistry was only just beginning. My sister and I used to be taken to Mumbai's famous and busy multi-speciality J.J. Hospital. I developed a fear of injections from the vitamin B injections I had as a child.

We were often sent off with the driver and maid to J.J. Hospital. From our home in the suburbs, as we drove to the hospital, we went past homes, markets, railway tracks, and people on the streets. Slowly, as we approached the hospital, we could only see the menacing, quiet stone walls of the mills. A huge, brown-grey chimney towered over a black flyover on which our car sped. The scene suddenly turned ominous and scary.

At the hospital, we walked through long corridors. I do not know whether we went past emergency or the orthopaedic department, but I recall seeing people on stretchers. Some were wounded and needed to be attended to, some were in fresh bandages turned red with blood. By the time we reached

146

the upper floors of the orthodontic department, I was totally panicked.

I remember one visit during which the doctor asked me to open my month and put in a cold metallic instrument in my month, and I screamed so loudly that the doctor's colleagues from the other rooms rushed in to ask what had happened. I still have a memory of the doctor looking sheepishly at his colleagues saying, "I only put this in her mouth." It was that harmless instrument with a round mirror on one end! I remember that, for me, the cold feel of the instrument is what instigated me to scream. Little wonder then that part of my treatment was done under general anaesthesia.

After I graduated from college, I was married off like all girls were in those days.

When I got pregnant, my doctor guided me to a gentle Canadian lady who had an infant and was teaching Lamaze breathing for labour, Mrs. Merry Wood.

I went to my natal home in Mumbai for my delivery. It was a tradition in our culture to go to your mother's home for the first delivery. I loved Mumbai, with its temperate climate and a wonderful culture of post-natal massages. Delhi had extreme dry summer and extreme dry and cold winter.

When labour began, I laboured at home for a day. I was admitted to the nursing home with contractions coming at 10-minute intervals. My doctor came to check me. He anticipated that the birth would take time and asked me whether it was okay if he went home for a while since it was his son's birthday. I readily agreed. My contractions were mild. I had no idea how long the process would take.

After he left, my mother suggested to me that I should walk. Since the room was quite small, I decided to walk in the corridor. Each time a contraction occurred, I stood against the wall and did my breathing. When it was gone, I resumed walking.

After a while I felt tired and felt like lying down, so I went back to my room. Suddenly a wave of anger surged forth in me, because my room did not have an attached bathroom. It made me so mad! Then it suddenly occurred to me that a negative mood swing is a sign of transition, a sign that birth should soon happen. I rang the call bell and said to the nurse, "I think I am about to deliver." She looked at me, mockingly smiled, and said, "If you were ready to deliver, you would be shouting and screaming," and off she went.

I asked myself, *Ok, how do I scream and shout?* Aloud I shouted, "Are you stupid? Are you idiotic? Do you not understand? I am telling you I am going to deliver."

Maybe to shut me up, the nurse came back and said she would check me. On checking me, she panicked. She could see the baby's head.

She rushed off to call the doctor, but the phone was dead. There were no mobile phones in those days. She then rushed to call the guard to fetch the doctor in a taxi, but the guard had gone to eat dinner. It was about 9pm.

Soon the resident doctor arrived. She was a sweet and gentle lady, Dr. D'souza. In a few pushes, the baby was born. It was a baby boy, with the cord around his neck. Thankfully, in 1975, there were no ultrasounds, so I had no anxiety built up in me about the cord being around the baby's neck. The baby was born peacefully, gently, in dim light and with no medication. I now realise what a perfect natural birth it was!

On being called a "good patient" after my easy labour, I was aghast! "How could I be a good patient?" I had been a nightmare for doctors. If I could be a good patient, anyone could be, likewise. The Lamaze breathing was magical indeed.

My baby was born in February, and my cousin was due in October. I told her all about the wonderful breathing and how it had been so helpful to me. I taught her the breathing.

When she started labour, I accompanied her and her mother to the hospital. As she had her contractions, I did effleurage for her – mild stroking of her lower abdomen.

As my aunt, her mother, watched, she said, "Forget about a job, this is what you should do" She knew I was searching for a job but was not able to land one. I had been to interviews and was searching.

I thought her statement was incredible. Was this a job I could do? I thought that my aunt had no idea what work meant. I could only think of work as going to an office from 9am to 5pm.

Soon, a dear friend got pregnant. I enthusiastically taught her the breathing method I had used. She too had an easy and natural childbirth.

Before I knew it, I was pregnant again with my second baby. By now I had become overconfident about the breathing method. Arrogantly, I thought to myself, "I know what needs to be done".

I went back to my doctor in Mumbai for my delivery. When labour began and I reached the nursing home, my doctor was at the other end of town. His instructions were, "She dilates very fast. Give her pethidine." When the nurse came with the injection, I said I did not want it. She rolled me over and jabbed me on my hip. After that injection, I felt woozy. I had to make an effort to do my breathing. Being overconfident, I had not practiced the breathing enough before this delivery as I should have. The breathing did help, but with considerable effort on my part.

The baby was born with the water bag intact and with a face presentation. The doctor burst the bag of water at birth. Yet again, thankfully ultrasounds were not commonly used then, so we had no idea that the baby was a face presentation until he was born.

Now, here I was, with two babies and still no job! My aunt's words rang back in my head. I visited my obstetrician in Delhi and said that if anyone enquired about learning breathing for labour, I could teach it.

After a few days, my obstetrician called, saying that a French lady wanted to learn about breathing for labour. She turned out to be a lovely lady, Mrs. Fovo, who also made a crazy statement similar to aunt. She pulled out a book written in French, which I could not read. She said I could write a book like that one. It was a book on pregnancy with some illustrations. I had very low esteem and thought to myself, "Me? Write a book?!" What a crazy idea!

For my birthday one year, I received a book on childbirth, printed by the National Childbirth Trust, London. (NCT). I was thrilled with the book and read it with interest. In those pre-internet days, I had no source of information or touch point to validate what I was teaching. My sister lived in London, and I asked her to find out how I could become an NCT teacher. She enquired for me and sent me details.

In the details were papers I needed to write upon the completion of my training. Since I had already been teaching, I felt I could write those papers. I filled out the papers and posted them to NCT, saying that I was a teacher from India and would like to train with them. They replied saying that Teacher's Panel would consider my case and get back to me.

That was followed by a long wait. Finally, since my sister lived in London, I went there. Contacting the NCT, I asked if I could train with them now that I was there. They were very welcoming. For about three months, I took part in activities, classes, workshops, and study days. I loved the NCT teachers.

They were warm and loving and offered so much wisdom and knowledge.

I also heard of and visited Janet Balska's Active Birth Center and Dr. Odent's unit at a hospital in Pithivers, France, where water birth was beginning to be practiced

Upon my return to Delhi, in 1981, under Dr. S.K. Bhandari's wing, I started to teach Mothercraft classes at Sir Gangaram Hospital.

Being in the hospital was a learning experience. My classroom was next to the labour room, and I often went in and out of the labour room, especially if one of my students was in labour. I learnt a lot about labour.

I revisited NCT in 1995, 1996, 2003, and 2012.

One day I received a letter from Chennai. The writer said he had heard that I taught how to handle labour and asked if I could help him and his wife. I said I could help and sent him handwritten notes with stick figures to explain posture and positions for labour. There was no Internet. The communication was conducted through the Indian Post office.

He asked how much he needed to pay, and I said 50 rupees. He sent me back a very nasty letter saying that I was cheating the public and many other hurtful things. I don't remember whether he sent any money at all, but what I do remember is the shame and embarrassment I felt.

I had the urge to help people, but I did not want to be shamed and blamed by them. I needed a neutral interface. I felt I needed to protect myself by being unreachable to them. I was wondering what to do. One day while reading the newspaper I saw an advertisement for Rupa Paperbacks.

Their books were modestly priced, within the amount of money women are given as shagan during festivals. One can loosely translate *shagan* as pocket money that women receive in festivals or auspicious occasions. That meant they could afford to buy themselves a Rupa Paperback without asking their husband or family for money.

I noted down the address of Rupa Paperbacks and visited their office. I met their editor, Mr. Nirupam Chatterjee. He listened to me and asked me to write a sample chapter, then another sample chapter. His critique was ruthless, but I did not mind, because I always felt that there was room for improvement.

Finally, the book was published in 1991, titled *Pregnancy*. I suddenly realised that my aunt's wish for me to do this work and Mrs. Fovo's suggestion I write a book had both come true!

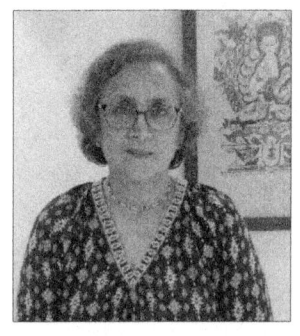 **Nutan L Pandit** has been teaching Birth Preparation classes since 1978. She has trained at National Childbirth Trust (NCT) London and is a National Trainer with Breastfeeding Promotion Network India (BPNI). She has authored three books, one of which has been translated into two languages. She has spoken at CME, Fortis Le Femme Hospital, Delhi; Fernandez Hospital, Hyderabad; Doordarshan TV and NDTV, and presented a paper at the Asia Pacific Midwifery Conference. She also practices complementary systems of healing. She's a Founding Member of Birthing The New Humanity.

Chapter 17

SOULBIRTH IN LOVE, NOT FEAR

By Faye Suzanne

Have you ever wondered why you are here, why you were born, and why certain things unfold the way they do in life? Sometimes life can be amazing… and other times not so, leaving you wondering what it's all about! In more recent times during the global pandemic, many people are living in fear, unsure if and when life will ever return to normal. Depression and suicide rates have increased, and the focus for improving mental health has become a high priority as people lose hope.

Given our current situation, we might be asking two big questions:

1. What is really happening on our planet at this time?

2. How can we navigate our way through these challenging times and not only survive, but thrive?

We are going through a time of great change here on Mother Earth. Not only is the earth herself changing and evolving to reach a higher vibrational frequency, but so too is all of humanity. Those souls choosing to incarnate at this time are bringing with them the frequencies to effect positive change on the planet.

Unfortunately, whenever great change is afoot, it is often preceded by a degree of chaos. That time is NOW. As unsettling as this change is, we WILL move through it. Nothing lasts forever. This too shall pass.

I liken the present time to the process of birth. Anyone who has ever given birth no doubt is familiar with that period just before birth occurs. We are so close, but at the point where we often lose our cool – it feels like it's never going to end. We feel ALL the sensations in our body and often relate it to pain and fear, as that is what we may have been conditioned to expect.

We may experience a disconnect from the birth process, our body, and often our mind. This period is known as transition. It is a natural phase of the birth cycle and is a wonderful message from our body that it is preparing for the birth. How amazing is that? At this point, we can choose whether we contract inward, holding onto the sensations increasing the intensity, or we can choose to ride the waves, much like surfing, to experience a joyful, ecstatic ride that floods us with endorphins (the feel-good hormones), leaving us feeling empowered. I know which one I'd choose every time, just as I did with the birth of each of my four children. For me, giving birth was the most incredibly powerful, spiritual, and enlightening experience of my life.

Each of my four births was completely different from the one before. They each offered me new insights to who I was as a person and opened me up to new ways of being and knowing. My second pregnancy and birth gave me an introduction to the more spiritual aspects of the journey and became pivotal in changing the way I view birth as a woman, as a mother, and as a midwife.

As a midwife of more than 34 years, I've had the privilege of witnessing new life enter into physicality thousands of times. It's such an honour to be present and to hold space for birthing couples and their babies and to bear witness to the miraculous event that is unfolding before me. I've always looked in wonder at newborn babies as I welcome them earthside, wondering what lies ahead of them on this journey and what gifts they are bringing with them to share with the world.

Not all births unfold in the way the parents have chosen, but I do believe **each birth unfolds in the way that was intended** for certain circumstances to play out for an experience to be shared or healing for all involved to take place. We are all spiritual beings having a physical experience, and we draw those experiences to us that will help us to grow and evolve. Growth can sometimes be painful, much like the transition phase of birth. How we choose to meet these circumstances will ultimately influence the quality of the experience and how we remember it.

Physical life is a journey that we each choose to take. We choose our parents, our place of birth, and our life situation – all of the elements that will help create the ideal environment for us to live our purpose, to express ourselves in the way we have chosen, and to help us to grow and evolve as a soul. It is not always easy, as we all have challenges along the way that we need to overcome. We are defined by how we show up on a daily basis and how we meet these challenges.

Throughout life, we will experience many different "births," not just that of ourselves or our babies. We give birth to ideas, to projects, and to new ways of being. We re-birth ourselves many times over in our lifetime, and each time, we go through similar stages to when we physically birth a baby.

First, we conceive the idea, project, a new way of being, etc. Sometimes the idea just drops in from nowhere, and other times we consciously conceive what it is we wish to birth into the world, whether physical or non-physical. When we consciously conceive, we can collaborate with our higher self, our soul, and other beings to bring clarity and vision to what is in alignment with our purpose and for our highest good. As with consciously conceiving a child, we can bring in all the elements to create a sacred space that provides a welcome landing space for the soul to enter. Whether this is by pure intent or by using physical tools such as crystals, essential oils, music, and sound, the important ingredient is the intention that lies behind it and the connection between the self, each other, and source or incoming soul.

Once conceived, the idea, project, or unborn baby will gestate, grow, and hopefully flourish, while bathing in the frequencies that are circulating in the "womb space." To give optimum conditions for healthy growth, we need to ensure that our frequencies are maintained at a high vibration. For instance, when a baby is growing in the womb, it is of utmost importance that we feed only positive, life-enhancing energy into the womb space. The baby is like a giant sponge and absorbs everything around it – nutrients, words, and energy. It is the same for our ideas, projects, and how we see ourselves in the world. If we feed ourselves negative thoughts, words, and intentions, these elements will manifest outwardly as a negative representation. However, if we feed positive, life-enhancing energy into these aspects, the results will be a positive outward expression of the self. Therefore, it is absolutely important that we feed ourselves, our unborn babies, and our ideas with only positive energy so we may experience positive results. Our babies blossom and grow healthy and strong when they are immersed in unconditional love and light, and they know that they are absolutely wanted, loved, and supported.

When growing my second baby in the womb, I became acutely aware of her soul around me. We were able to communicate with one another very clearly, and I got to know her on a deep level. She would communicate about what she wanted and needed before she was born and direct me in the healing I needed to undergo both personally and together with her. She called in my birth team and told me what she wanted well before she was born. I found a deep sense of connection with her, which I still feel today, 29 years later. Under my daughter's guidance, she was born underwater in a free-standing birth centre, in the caul, blessed to be surrounded by those who deeply loved and wanted her. It was an otherworldly experience; her soul had been guiding me through the whole process. She was my spiritual midwife. This gave me a new perspective on what physical birth is all about from the soul's perspective. This then led me down the rabbit hole of spiritual birth and how to help facilitate it for others. It changed me in so many wonderful ways and on so many different levels.

The deepening continued as I journeyed through pregnancy loss, health concerns, and two more amazing and deeply spiritual births. Each experience taught me more and called me to dive deeper and deeper into the unknown, meeting many of my fears head on. As my understanding grew with each new experience, I overcame my fears and learned to lean into them, breathing my way through until I emerged on the other side with a more expanded view.

As the time for any birth approaches, we often begin nesting and preparing ourselves physically, mentally, emotionally, and spiritually. Our senses are heightened at this time, and our intuition strengthens. This time is so important, as it offers us the opportunity to go within and to connect with ourselves, our baby, and a higher source and come to know that everything will be okay. Even if things become chaotic for a while or we experience loss or devastation, our inner knowing and our connection to a higher source will guide us through, if we allow it.

As we journey through birth, we have a choice to show up in fear and contraction or love and expansion. The first time we take this path, it is relatively unknown, which can be very daunting. Even though I was already a midwife when I first experienced a birth of my own, it was completely different from what I expected. I knew the process theoretically and physically, as I'd supported other women through it hundreds of times already. But to embody birth is a completely different experience. To connect with the sensations in my body and to feel how it responded to this process was interesting, to say the least. I had an intense but very empowering birth that gave me a whole new appreciation for the women I cared for as they birthed their babies.

After the birth, a new journey began. Not only had my baby emerged into physical life, but I had also emerged as a mother. I had been reborn with a new identity and new experiences to navigate. There were some common threads and recognisable aspects of the me that existed before, but somehow I had changed. The continuum of birth, life, death, and rebirth kicked into action as a conscious awareness of self. I realised as I was taken deeper into my spiritual journey that this is what we are here to experience: life itself, in its ever-changing, ever-expanding nature. We are here to experience it all – the good, the bad and all the in-between spaces. All of it is valuable and exciting when we can see it for what it is, not just the emotional attachment to the illusion that is playing out in the present moment.

When we can relate all of the above to what is happening at the present time, we can see that Mother Earth is rebirthing herself. She is currently in her transition phase and, as such, is contracting and expanding to allow changes to take place. Humanity is largely reacting out of fear, as they are uncomfortable with this phase of the birth process, much like I have witnessed in the birthing space over many years.

We are being called to work through our fears, our pain, and our trauma, to acknowledge that which no longer resonates deep within us and trust our intuition, now more than ever. This is so that we can support this mama to rebirth herself into a space of love, NOT fear, as that will determine how she grows and evolves into the future. Just think of the energy you would like to have in the space that you choose to experience your birth. Would you choose a space filled with fear and drama or of love and support? Which energy is more conducive to growth, expansion, and joy? What frequency of energy do we as a human family wish to bathe in as we co-exist with Mother Earth and one another? It is a choice. Whichever we choose, we will attract all others that vibrate at the same frequency into our field. Imagine a world where humanity has chosen love over fear. Our collective consciousness would then emanate this energy to all other lifeforms around us and the planet. This, I believe, is our mission. **To BE love. This is our natural state.**

Through love, we can let go of fear and heal our trauma, no matter what form it takes, and change our beliefs about ourselves and others. If we can do this, our world will be changed for the better.

After working with women and couples for more than 30 years to help heal their birth trauma and re-frame birth, I know that we CAN heal, grow, and thrive, each and every one of us, no matter our age or life experience. We just have to say YES and remember that we are spiritual beings, and we were all born to thrive. Mother Earth needs us to heal ourselves so that we can show up fully conscious to support her as she re-births herself.

Are you in?

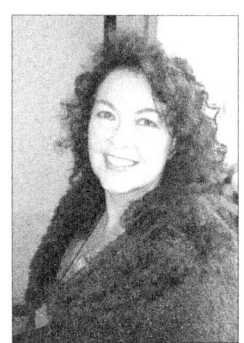 **Faye Suzanne** is a Midwife for the New Humanity. Her Soul Calling is to remind others of their true nature and the journey they chose to take as humans. Her greatest teachers have been the four amazing souls that she was honoured to bring earthside. She is also a proud grandmother of three cheeky boys. Her 34 years' experience as a midwife and a lifetime of working with energy and Spirit birthed the concept of Soulbirth.

Chapter 18

OUT OF TRAUMA, BACK TO HAPPINESS

By Jutta Wohlrab

Starting Out

I was born in a small clinic on a beautiful morning in May 1963 to delighted parents. My father was unusual for his time in having attended the births of all three of his children. My mother would revisit the story of my birth every year (on my birthday, of course!), and she would always finish by saying, 'Your birth was something special. It was such an easy birth, and you came into the world looking around with big eyes as if you wanted to see and understand everything."

This story has stayed with me and probably explains why, after nursing ambitions to be a journalist, an actor, and an artist, I decided at the age of 16 or 17 (and already a dedicated feminist and humanist) to become a midwife. I didn't actually know any midwives, anything about the job at all, or even any pregnant women, but I knew I would enjoy working with people. In what other profession, I reasoned, could you make a difference in the very beginning of someone's life and champion the rights of women and girls? I had made up my mind, and nothing – not even the fierce competition for placement at midwifery schools – was going to stop me. I was a born optimist, determined not only to maintain a positive spirit, but also to share it with the world.

I gathered as much information as I could and went to the bookshop to see what I could find on the subject. The very first book I picked up was Frederick Leboyer's groundbreaking *Birth Without Violence*. His focus on the baby's awareness from the earliest days in the womb and on natural childbirth resonated with me and confirmed for me that I had chosen the right career.

It has to be said that the 1970s and 1980s were dark days for the craft of midwifery, but luckily, the only school out of the many I applied to that offered me a place was one that worked according to Leboyer's principles. So began my journey into the heart of the most miraculous event a woman will ever experience.

That was over three decades ago. Since then, I have welcomed over 3,000 babies into the world and supported over 10,000 women. I have worked in all kinds of settings, from home births, to birthing centres, to labour wards in large teaching hospitals, across two continents, gathering perspectives on birth from a range of cultures. I now share my knowledge as an international expert at international conferences, through podcasts and television, writing articles, and last but not least through online courses and workshops.

What inspired me from the start – and still inspires me every day – was the quest to provide every woman with a positive experience. How was it, I used to wonder, that one woman could just come in and give birth naturally and easily, while another could have such pain and difficulty? For me, every birth was an opportunity to understand this conundrum and to gain insight into how I could resolve the problems mothers encountered.

I began to understand how seriously fears, worries, and the shadow of long-past trauma could impact the process of childbirth. Take Ulrike, for example: her first child had been born with a genetic disorder, and though she and her husband loved their daughter dearly, they knew they would not be able to care for another child with such serious needs. Genetic testing revealed no problems, and the pregnancy proceeded smoothly. The early stages of labour went well, but when it was time to push, Ulrike suddenly held back, afraid that history would repeat itself. I encouraged her to breathe, to accept that what would be would be, and to say "yes" to the new baby. She did so, and a beautiful baby boy emerged into the world.

Aligning Body and Mind

Ulrike had demonstrated to me the power that our minds can have over our bodies. I began to encounter more and more women who had experienced traumatic life events in previous births or who had simply developed a fear of childbirth. It got me thinking that I wanted to empower these women and support them.

Wouldn't it be great if every woman could feel confident about the capacity of her body to deliver a baby? Shouldn't everyone involved in the birth be able to look back on a glorious event? That became my goal for every pregnancy and birth I attended. I decided to become an NLP trainer and a hypnotherapist.

What is needed for a good birth is not only a deep understanding of the physiological processes at work, but also control over your mind and alignment with the body. I went on to embrace all of the disciplines that I felt promoted this fruitful union of mind and body, so I also trained in acupuncture and as a yoga teacher, developing ante-natal and post-natal yoga courses.

These techniques came to the fore when I worked with Beate. She had been sexually abused as a child, but now had met a loving man, gotten married, and became pregnant. Her biggest fear about the forthcoming birth was that if anything went wrong, the midwife could end up with having to call in male specialists. Our NLP work together did much to help her feel happier and more confident.

She was therefore well equipped to cope when, during labour, the baby's heart rate gave rise to concern. She went deep within herself, to her mental safe place, using all the techniques she had learnt, and eventually gave birth standing up. Although the baby was fine, Beate herself was bleeding heavily, and the midwife was obliged to call on a male colleague – Beate's worst nightmare. However, the consultant's gentle, respectful examination of her, combined with support from the inner resources we had worked on, turned this experience into one of profound healing.

She came to me again during her second pregnancy to prepare for the birth with yoga, acupuncture, and hypnobirthing, but now she was confident, joyful, and secure in the knowledge that she was strong and in control.

Healing from Trauma

My quest never ceases. I am always open to discovering and investigating new practices that can help us, and I have recently added eye movement desensitisation programming (EMDR) and brainspotting (a method of tackling trauma through identifying certain eye positions).

I became convinced of the effectiveness of these techniques in the aftermath of a visit to Kathmandu, during which I experienced an earthquake. People's lives were changed, including mine, in the course of 90 seconds. After the earthquake hit, people in the centre of the city were running and screaming, shops I had visited only hours before had been transformed into rubble, and bodies lay strewn around the market square.

I helped out in Nepal as much as I could for two weeks but finally returned to Germany, where I had a complete meltdown. As luck would have it (or was it pre-ordained?), I was due to go on an advanced NLP training session on – of all things – trauma. During the training, every time I talked about my experience of the earthquake in front of thirty other people, I became very emotional, dissolving into tears, for some reason overwhelmed with guilt that I hadn't done more to help in Nepal. I was fortunate that my teacher worked with me using EMDR, and to my amazement, after only a few sessions over the course of two days, I was restored to my previous happy and joyful self. But I am also a practical person, and now I have found another technique through which I could bring more positivity and healing to the world.

It is only now, I think, that the true impact of trauma in all its forms is being recognised more widely. Its effect on the women I have worked with over the years has been very obvious. In these days of Zoom calls and consultations, I often think of Rasia.

Rasia found me through a Facebook group. She had only been in Germany for a year and did not speak any German, only a little English. This meant that she had been unable to explain her misgivings about her pregnancy when she visited the doctor at 35 weeks and had had no option but to accept his reassurance that everything was fine. But at her next visit, at 36 weeks, no heartbeat was detected, and she had been obliged to deliver her stillborn baby alone in a foreign country, without the support of family or friends. Again, her lack of German prevented her from taking up any of the help offered by the hospital.

It was a year after this sad event that she contacted me. We talked about everything that had happened, and she cried and cried. I offered to work with her, and after our first session, she sent me a message saying, "This is the first time after twelve months that I've slept free of nightmares and been able to go out shopping." After a few more sessions, she was able to travel and go to visit her family in Jordan, which was a big step. Laughter and joy returned to her life, and in a few months, she got a job. A year after our first meeting, she was pregnant again, and this time gave birth to a healthy baby.

The Foundation of Our Lives

My life has been full of stories like these, and I love to tell them. But no matter the different details, the essence of them is always healing. You could almost say that the process of birth itself needs healing, because it is a natural function from which we have distanced ourselves in many cultures. The evidence is clear to see in the prevalence of C-sections globally, the highest rate ever of birth interventions, the anxieties of pregnant women, and the level of post-natal depression.

Life starts in the womb. How a prospective mother feels makes a difference in how a baby feels. Pregnancy should be a creative time filled with love, happiness, and connectedness. It's my mission to support that in whatever way I can, whether by helping release trauma and preparing the way for a smooth delivery or by giving people the knowledge they need to get the birthing experience they want. Knowledge is empowerment.

Modern technology has enabled us to connect in different ways, and the pandemic has certainly accelerated this process. I never tire of sharing my knowledge with people all over the world, and it is a privilege to combine my medical expertise with my experience in a range of holistic therapies in the workshops and courses that I run for an international audience. It may be a long process, but I feel that I am helping to bring about a quiet revolution in attitudes towards birth.

In the words of the old song, we need to "accentuate the positive." Every day of your pregnancy that is a good day tilts the balance in favour of positivity. In fact, whether you're pregnant or not, asking yourself the following four questions and writing down the answers will help you to do that.

- What gave me joy today?
- When did I feel alive today?
- Who and what can I be grateful for today?
- Which of my strengths was I able to draw on today?

I am truly grateful to all of the women whose stories I will carry with me forever and for everything I have learned from them and will continue to learn. I leave you with the following observation from the great birth pioneer Sheila Kitzinger:

"Childbirth takes place at the intersection of time; in all cultures it links past, present, and future. In traditional cultures, birth unites the world of now with the world of the ancestors and is part of the great tree of life extending in time and eternity."

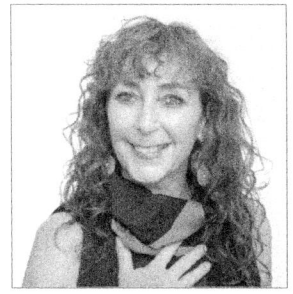

Jutta Wohlrab is an enthusiastic and inspiring midwife, coach, trainer, bestselling author, and international speaker with over 38 years of experience. She enjoys traveling the world to share her knowledge and experience. Based in Berlin, she works online and offline with international clients. Her vision is that women all over the world should have a joyful, safe, and happy birth. Find out more about her courses at www.juttawohlrab.com and via social media.

Chapter 19

SOUL BIRTH

How we change the world by remembering our birth and who we truly are

By JoAnn Lowell

"One of the most calming and powerful actions you can do to intervene in a stormy world is to stand up and show your soul. Soul… shines like gold in dark times."
~ Clarissa Pinkola Estes

The darkest part of the crisp March night is completely still. At this hour, there are no "fietsen" bicycles ringing their bells as they zing over the canal bridges. We are in a softly lit birthing room in an Amsterdam clinic, sitting in quietude on the edge of time. A new soul is arriving to the earth on this clear night.

I am here as a Canadian architecture student doing research for my thesis, "The Place of Birth." In the 1980s, the Netherlands is renowned for the lowest infant and maternal mortality rates in the world, with half their births at home and half in hospital. In the birthing room, I am facing the mother, dutifully drawing her, the room, the bed, her husband, and midwife, as I take in all of the environmental factors. This process lasts for 20 minutes before I throw my sketchbook to the floor.

I am overcome by the instinct to breathe every breath with this new mother. As she breathes in, I breathe in. As she breathes out, I breathe out. Long, slow breaths in together… out together. Our eyes are locked in a place of No Time. Something deep inside of me is awakened. I reach deep down inside, and I remember that I am a midwife. Every fibre of my being knows this. My soul knows this. We breathe this way facing each other long into the night.

At the break of dawn, a new soul arrives. This new mother squats on the floor as her son gushes forth, born into her arms to triumphant cries of joy. At this moment, a morning star rises. The first blackbird faces the eastern sky and sings to the golden dawn and to this new baby. He is a one-of-a-kind soul, a unique piece of this puzzle of humanity, just like this moment is unique across the entire universe, never to be repeated again in exactly this way. The whole universe joins in a welcoming chorus at each and every moment of birth.

On that night in Amsterdam, I remember who I am. My soul knows what it knows, and when I follow it, it sings. Birth discovered me, and I answered the call.

~ * ~

An ancient Buddhist story tells of an old blind turtle who lives at the bottom of the vast ocean. In the middle of this vast ocean floats a single piece of driftwood with a hole in the middle of it. It is tossed from wave to wave by the rolling water. Every hundred years, the old turtle swims to the surface for a breath of air. It is said that when the turtle reaches the surface, the likelihood that his head will find the hole in the driftwood is greater than the likelihood of being incarnated as a human.

The greatest invitation to our soul's growth is to incarnate within a human life. I am grateful for mine and for yours.

In the adventure of my human life, my architectural thesis took me around the globe into many birth cultures. Out of this came my love of birth, where I came into my calling as a traditional birth attendant (midwife) in the Indigenous communities where I lived and practiced in the high Arctic. Along the way, I received many teachings:

- We don't know until we step out of the particular birth culture we are living in that it has positive and negative influences on us. Know that we can step out of it. We can change our cultures.
- One of the greatest, simplest, and oldest of human technologies runs through all birth cultures and all of our lives. It is right under our noses: the power of our conscious breath. This is the vessel we ride through every heightening wave and ebbing flow of birth.
- We come to earth and experience our first breath. When we leave our bodies at the end of our earth walk, we release our last breath. The Ojibway people have a name for all the breaths in between: *Misganou.*

Conscious Breathing

Through my work with birthing, I was awakened to a deep love of the extraordinary power of conscious breathing, and I trained as a professional Breathwork Practitioner. How we breathe from our first to our last breath matters. It shows us how to soulfully move through life's ups and downs, through our thoughts and feelings, and through the chaos and calm of our gorgeous, messy human lives.

The allegorical sensation of conscious breathing, of birthing, and of life shows up in our bodies. You can try this:

EXPANSION – On the inhale, breathe deeply down into your belly and pelvis. Fill your chest. Feel your ribs and back expanding.

CONTRACTION – Fully release on the long exhale. Feel your whole body relax, especially your jaw, neck, and shoulder muscles. Let go.

MOVEMENT – Notice with each breath that you are inching toward a destination (...a destiny?) You cannot see it, yet you sense it.

When guided through conscious, connected breathing, we are able to gently move through and heal trauma which is somatically lodged in our bodies. This lights up our soul and turns our shadows into gold when we integrate it.

> "There is a crack, a crack in everything.
> That's how the light gets in."
> ~ Rumi

Conscious breathing is so simple and accessible that I train teachers and parents to teach daily exercises to children starting as young as 3 years old, all the way up to high school and university. Children can be taught how to feel and safely regulate their bodies and emotions. From a young age, they come to realize that the soul of the universe is in them, and now they see it in everyone and everything around them.

Birth Imprints

I asked myself this question a long time ago: What if we went through birth consciously and gently with deep, inner preparation for our souls entering into this human life, using all of these tools in our healing satchel?

During breathwork sessions, I came to witness that we often remember our births and our past lives. My work begins with mothers- and fathers-to-be starting with their own arrival to earth. We examine how the imprints from their own births can predispose their ways of relating and unconsciously affect their lives. From my experience, I am aware that our birth imprints are especially alive for each one of us at every birth.

From a soul perspective, part of our job is to "make friends" with these birth imprints for the unique lessons and gifts they bring. They can show up in small, nuanced ways or in big ways in our behaviours, while they almost always arise from our unconscious self. For example, someone who is born breech (feet or bum first) may seem to be going the opposite direction of others in the river of life. This may get them into situations at odds with others. The lesson their soul came to receive may be to learn that having a different way is not cause for alienation. The gift of their soul's unique way of seeing things upside down may often be the stroke of genius to envision new things from a fresh perspective.

I witness that people who are born prematurely can often be early to appointments, and those of us born late are often late. That describes one aspect of my birth! I was always anxiously late, yet no amount of time management coursework could change this until I acknowledged my own birth imprints. That's when I came to learn that I flow on God's Time. Aha!

Folks with easy births may look for more difficult challenges in their lives. A person with a Caesarean-section birth may not understand all the methodical steps of manifesting a project. When there are difficult conditions in a pregnant mother's life, the baby may grow up to see themselves having to put other people's needs first before their own. These experiences can become the gift of learning to embody compassion for ourselves and for others.

My experience suggests to me that many obstetricians likely had a near-death experience at their birth. They can unconsciously have a need to save lives, even with normal, healthy birthing women. Without saying a word, during a birth I slide up next to the obstetrician. I take three audibly deep and long breaths. By the third breath, they are breathing slow and deep to the breathing rhythm I've introduced. Without fail, they suddenly look up and are softly jolted back into the present moment. The trance of the impact of their birth imprint is broken.

I knew from the beginning that if we change the way we birth, we change the world. During pregnancy, I work with both mothers and fathers on the impact of their own deep-rooted birth imprints through somatic breathwork, emotional release, and guided visualizations and affirmations. Consistently we see this work can completely change birthing outcomes or the need for interventions.

In the throes of birth, when a detour happens, the journey forward is not what we thought it would be. I regularly witness everyone's birth imprints are activated. Almost everyone involved goes into chaos and often forgets the mother.

At this point in time, we can't push the river back. I then announce, "All is well. There is another soul in the room. What if this is exactly what this new soul needs for their incarnation here on earth?" To the mother I say, "Your love is so great, you are giving this new soul the exact birth they need for the lessons they came to learn and the gifts they came here to share. What I know for sure is that every birth is perfect."

We snap out of the trance of our own birth imprints or "what if" and suddenly remember we are souls within the greater universal pattern. In these times of experiencing chaos, the soul can light up the alignment of priorities for our life's task.
We come to accept that there were no mistakes with our births, only gifts and lessons for the soul. Our imperfections are a big part of our perfection from the soul's point of view. All the soul wants to do is evolve.

Ancestors

The act of birthing, just like dying, is the greatest threshold we will cross. The ancestors are especially present at the moment of birth and at death, showering us with their love. Many – even most – Indigenous cultures believe the ancestors are present here and now and live within each of us as a promise written upon our hearts. When I nap during a long birth, I have dreamed that there are other family members of the birthing family who are present. I will ask them, "Who is this woman I dreamed of?" The answer will be, "That is my mother who just died – she is the grandmother of this new babe." Of course she is here.

In a small hamlet in the Canadian Arctic, I was introduced to an Inuit belief that the last person in the family to die is the one who is being born in this moment now. To them, this is one continuous cycle where there is no separation between life and death and birth. If Grandpa had the most recent death, the family calls out "Grandpa Charlie" when the birth is imminent. Even if the child born is female, they will name her Charlie, they will dress her in Grandpa's clothes, and give her his pipe. Most importantly, they will treat her with the respect of an Elder from the moment of her birth and throughout her life.

This echoes the well-known story of the Dalai Lama, who was trained in each lifetime to remember who he is. When he was age 2 and correctly identified all of his personal possessions from his previous incarnation, he was recognized as the 14th Dalai Lama. At age 15, he was the leader of Tibet and faced the threat of an imminent invasion from the Chinese army. He meditated all night. When he emerged the next morning, he remembered he is the incarnation of all 13 previous Dalai Lamas going back to 1391 CE. He recognized that he knew how to face this moment with the Chinese army, because he had done it many times before.

In turbulent times, we can draw upon the strength and wisdom of our own earlier incarnations. We can know we are the answered prayers of our ancestors. They live through us and are present in every breath of the newborn child.

~ * ~

One day God ponders this riddle: I am God, but how do I truly know I am God? S/He decides to do an experiment. We human souls as spirit are sent to Earth with an inner divine spark of

God within us. There is a catch. Upon our arrival, we won't remember we are God. The experiment is intended for us to ask throughout the journey of our lives what is God and what is not God so that we can know the difference. That way, we will truly know what is God.

Over time, I came to question this story. In fact, I believe we come to discover that everything is God (or Spirit or the Great Mystery). Everyone, everything, and every experience belongs; there is nothing that is separate. I pondered that this original hypothetical experiment from God has gone sideways. One of the greatest tragedies is that we have forgotten who or what we truly are.

Then an idea came to me: what if we simply started at the moment of birth to stop forgetting? What if we just remember our true self from the beginning, and we continue to remember this all the days of our lives? I teach each new parent these words that I say to every new soul on the day of their birth:

"You remember who you are. You remember why you came. You will always remember this. You are a beautiful Child of God. You will always remember who you are."

For Our Times
In this stormy world in this challenging era, it helps to know that:
- Birth becomes the metaphor for the times we are living in.
- Breath becomes the metaphor for the way through.
- Change is the one constant in this life.
- We have learned how to navigate the changes in our lives.
- Through our own births, we came through the biggest transition just fine.

During challenges, just like with birth:
Trust the process. Stay with it, even when there is discomfort. It will not last forever. None of us move through life without pain

as a part of the human experience. The key is learning to stay present with it and trust that it has a purpose.

Find yourself in the calm in the middle of the storm. Bring yourself out of your mind at the top of the tree and down into your roots. Breathe here. Breathe into your heart. Be the source of peace to yourself and to all those around you. Breathe. And trust the river has a destination.

> "For each child that's born,
> a morning star rises and sings
> to the universe who we are…
> We are ONE."
> ~ Ysaye M. Barnwell, Sweet Honey in the Rock

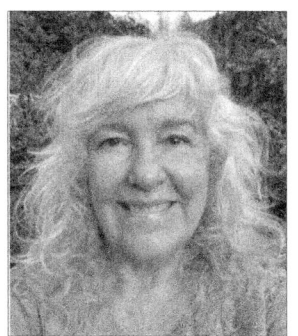 **JoAnn Lowell** is a warm and captivating international speaker, a Traditional Birth Attendant, and a professional Breathwork Practitioner. The founder of Soul Medicine, she has been a visionary for the International Breathwork Foundation and many organizations. Her work as the creator of Conscious Breathing in the Classroom has gone to the UN. She is aligned with wisdom teachings from the Indigenous communities where she lives on the unceded land of the Sinixt in Canada.

SoulMedicine.One

Chapter 20

EMBRACING THE CHILD OF THE WOMB: A MIDWIFE'S' JOURNEY

By Irene Chain Kalinowski

Introduction

Life is a journey, and crossing the turbulent streams to follow my dreams has been the most amazing rollercoaster ride that one could ever imagine. It has encompassed relationships, friendships, family, health, wealth, work, creativity, courage, and confidence to speak out to people close to me and on the public stage.

What has life in the womb got to do with any of the above? What has spirituality got to do with it?

The answer is EVERYTHING. Looking back on my entire journey so far, I can clearly see the jigsaw puzzle coming together. It is almost complete. If only I knew more about it at a young age, it wouldn't have taken 65 years to get to this point.

How can my journey help you? You won't have to wait 65 years; you can start right now to help yourself and do the right thing for your newborn child.

My life in my mother's womb – afraid to speak out.

I learned the hard way that just about all of my failures had something to do with what I was exposed to as I was growing in my mother's womb.

As a child I was quite shy, very smart, but very sensitive. I didn't want to say anything that might hurt someone, and I would never put my hand up in class for fear of getting it wrong. When I tried playing netball, I wasn't even strong enough to get the ball.

If someone made any sensitive remarks about my clothes or my body, I would get very bad cramps in my bowel. When I was a teenager, I endured many bowel issues, such as constipation. The doctors gave me plenty of laxatives and told my parents it was hereditary. Eventually I developed a spastic bowel, and during surgery, the doctors removed all but one foot of it. I couldn't understand why I didn't feel any better afterward, and for years, I continued to struggle with related health issues.

In 1995, I arrived in New Zealand, marking a turning point in my life. New Zealand was a spiritual country, and the residents are open to many natural therapies.

I came across a homeopath named Sally. We had a two-hour session, during which she covered subjects like my life, my relationships, my dreams, my parents, the foods I liked and disliked, and of course my physical issues.

Sally presented the following issues to explain my health problems:

My parents were war refugees from Poland. My mother faced extensive trauma during the war. They had to keep many secrets and were afraid to speak out. My mother carried all of this post-war stress trauma and passed it on to me whilst she was pregnant.

This manifested as:

- Fear to speak out.
- Sensitivity to others.
- Sensitivity to others' remarks.
- Acceptance of mental abuse.
- Fear of someone looking over one's shoulder.

Sally gave me a homeopathic medicine to match my entire being. I took that energetic medicine, and I felt everything lift. The words I couldn't say came flowing out, and energetically it was as if I had been elevated onto a spiritual plane.

From there, I never looked back. I took elocution lessons and lessons in the power of speech. Today I find it so easy to take the stage with confidence and without fear of anyone looking over my shoulder. I am never afraid to say what I need to say. If I met Sally 20 years prior, I would still have my bowel, but I also would not have been able to share this story with you.

I received many good qualities from my parents also. I had a very loving environment. My parents were very compassionate and caring for others. They had a love for music, and my pregnant mother danced at many Polish parties. They also had a gift for accounting, and I grew to be very clever at math, and no one could ever keep me off the dance floor.

I studied homeopathy and incorporated it into my midwife practice. Today I have used it for 20 years to help women sustain a happy and healthy pregnancy. It also helps in removing negative blocks. During their pregnancies, I encourage women and their partners to take time to communicate and connect with their beautiful baby who is thriving and growing in the womb. I know how truly important the connection between the pregnant woman and early development of the baby is, because I have personally experienced the psychological and physical suffering from its negative impact.

Childbirth as a spiritual event.

My midwifery experience has taken me through four continents. I wish I could have cried tears of joy than of sadness, but the truth is that women are so fearful of childbirth. Many have surrendered and become accustomed to birthing in a medicalized environment, with interventions and the belief that this is the norm. They have lost the trust in the capabilities of their own divine body.

My grandmother had 13 children, all birthed at home. She was the village "baby catcher" in Poland. She used to share her stories with me. I asked her, "Did you see many women die in childbirth?" She said "None."

My mother birthed four of us at home. Although my sisters had their first babies in hospital, they refused to go back because of the all-too-prevalent interventions, and they subsequently had their children at home.

My great nieces surrendered to modern ways and developed complications of pregnancy; each had a cesarean section. Their children were unsettled and sick, and Autism appeared for the first time in our family. It was all there, staring at me in the face. Whilst I ventured throughout the world sharing my knowledge and experience assisting mothers give birth, childbirth itself was becoming a monetary event. I learned:

Medical hospitals rose from the floor.
Homebirths are not encouraged anymore.
Oops did the doctors omit to wash their hands?
Women and babies died…Infection rates soared.
Florence Nightingale cleansed the wards.
Ensured sterile environments, masks, gowns and gloves.
Removing compassion and love.
Women's perceptions that doctors must attend births are now here to stay.
Midwife skills lost and a thing of the past.

Women became mild and compliant.
Invalids who needed a servant.
"Oh doctor, tell me what to do!"
"I can't do this without you!"
The woman would not say she had labor beginning.
She would say, 'Doctor, I am SICK, the baby is coming!!!!'

Medical dominance continued to surge.
Medically assisted pain free birth began to emerge.
Visit Tombstone and you will see, on row four:
"Mrs. Stumpf died in childbirth, an overdose of chloroform, in
1884."
Strict asepsis and twilight sleep
brought women to the hospital to receive medical treats.
Out of its feelings, baby arrives gasping for air.
An increasing demand for those French "resuscitaires"
Sleepy babies unable to attach to the breast.
Dehydration and jaundice, the spin-off effect.
Baby's whisked away under pediatric care.
The new mother alone and in despair.
Formula promoted to be the best.
Children's Immune systems became weak and stressed
Separated from their mother's chest.

It is understandable why women fear birth; I feared it as a very young midwife. That's because I didn't understand it. Yet with observation and learning from women about the process, delving deep into its mysteries, fear ended, and I could no longer be kept from attending a birth.

Women can do that, too, if they take the time to learn about it. When they understand the process and what is happening and connect with their baby, they become confident, reaping the rewards of an uncomplicated, normal, and spiritual birth. When you do all of the above, you stay in control. Take it from me: the loss of control can lead to a lifetime of depression, physical illness, and regret. Babies are more content and healthier when birthed without fear.

It's simple: eat healthy foods, exercise, reduce stress, remove negativity, connect with your body and your baby, and grow a baby proportionate in size to you.

Birth story

Annie had had two normal, uncomplicated births with her first partner. Life got complicated, and the relationship with her partner ended. She met someone new and had two babies via C-section with her new partner.

She came to me with her 5th pregnancy.

I reviewed her cesarian history. It was clear to see she had not received any counselling or holistic advice. Her partner, Pete, had not been present for the birth of the babies by C-section. It was clear that these occurred due to stress and a cascade of interventions, but this time, they wanted a vaginal birth.

I counselled both of them. Annie had suffered abuse in her childhood and faced many unresolved issues. Pete had suffered mental abuse from his family as they had excessive expectations of him.

I gave them homeopathic remedies to remove their negative blocks, a combination of Staphysagria, Ignatia, and Natrum muriaticum. They both felt lighter and uplifted towards a spiritual plane with the remedies. I armed them with videos about self-care, preparing for birth, and the birth.

It was New Year's Day when Annie went into labor. I lived at least an hour away. Peter came to collect me, and I spent the entire day with them. We had lunch, and I entertained the children. Peter and Annie nurtured each other, I did nothing, and the labor progressed. We could see the baby move and descend abdominally. I knew there was no need for intervention.

Eventually I could see Annie was holding back. She took some more homeopathic remedies.

She asked me to examine her, so I did. The baby was ready to come, but her emotions held on, and with a little tough love I said, "You have a pelvis like a bucket, and your baby wants to come out!" With that she relaxed and birthed a beautiful baby boy in a quiet, peaceful, and loving environment. She placed her baby skin to skin. The little boy found his way to the breast and fed without any help. Peter lay right beside her, looking at them in awe.

The placenta took a little time to come, so Peter placed baby skin to skin whilst Annie stood up and delivered her placenta naturally.

We took a family photo with the children. A million dollars could not replace the love and cries of joy that came from the couple. "I won't have any more children, but I will remember this day for the rest of my life." Annie said, hugging me. I felt 10 years younger because of the joy. This was the end and a new beginning, the release of trauma for the parents and a beautiful new beginning for this little boy.

That is how birth should be.

The Newborn

Babies who have been birthed vaginally without interventions always seem to be more content. The postpartum period seems to be a breeze for mothers who are self-aware of themselves and who have connected with their baby during the pregnancy.

It's a very different story for babies who are born to mothers who have had interventions during birth, or via a C-section. Most of these mothers carry their pre-pregnancy negativities with them. Anxieties lead to many physical problems for the new mother and the newborn baby.

- Baby's refuse the breast.
- Startle in their sleep.
- Fail to feed and thrive.
- Have more colic.

I treat many of these inconsolable babies with homeopathy. One doesn't need to be a scientist to explain this, as I have witnessed it for the last 40 years. Old wise women used to say that a baby will pick up the mother's emotions during pregnancy and during the postpartum period. Newborn babies have feelings. Babies who have been separated from their mothers and nursed in incubators carry lifelong feelings of abandonment. Many grow up to become parents themselves and detach themselves from their own children. Homeopaths treat many cases like this.

My role in the new spiritual world

For 40+ years, I have witnessed that our global modern corporate systems fail women and their families and that women are not educated or supported with a preventative holistic model that embraces the mind-body-earth connection.

My cat gave birth to 8 kittens on my bed. No one told her what to do. She birthed the kittens, they found their way to the breast, the placenta was delivered, she ate it, and she even cleaned up after it.

"Why can't humans do that?" Well, they can, but they need to be in a safe and loving environment, and they need to be in tune with mother nature.

Today I sit on the international stage, sharing experiences and teaching women and midwives how to embrace birth. My new role is that of Head of Midwifery Council for the Wakaminenga Health Council here in New Zealand.

We are preparing for a new education platform that is based on *Whakaako Te Pepi o Te Whare Tangata*: "Teaching the child of the womb." It is aimed at creating a dynamic in which learning happens before the child is born into this world. The education for midwifery training and that of women and families also promotes the notion that healthy and confident mothers make healthy babies, and that birth is a spiritual event.

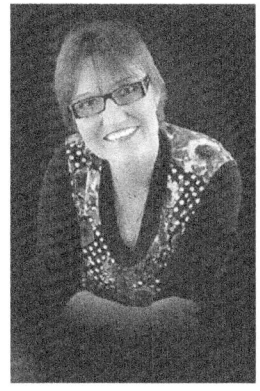

Irene Chain Kalinowski currently lives in New Zealand. She has practiced midwifery for 40+ years and has worked in Europe, The Middle East, China, and New Zealand. She has practiced homeopathy for 20 years. Irene lectures internationally and has authored many books, such as *My Body, My Baby, The Heart and Soul of Midwifery, With Woman, with Midwife, with Me, Three Blind Mice – A Midwife's Tale*, and *How Birth Was, How It Is, and How It Should Be*. She has also authored many midwifery textbooks based on an integrated holistic model of maternity care.

Chapter 21

MIDWIFES – AGENTS OF CHANGE

By Dr. Evita Fernandez

Let's rewind a bit to when I was eight. I knew I wanted to be a doctor, and I had absolutely no other profession in my mind. By the time I was 16, I knew I wanted to be an obstetrician. I wanted to take care of women who were pregnant and help them through birthing their babies.

I guess this came from the fact that my mother was an obstetrician and set up a hospital with two beds. At supper time, we would meet with my siblings and my parents. She would talk about her experiences with so much joy and fire in her. I thought, "Wow. This sounds great."

When I finished my house surgery, I was attracted to birthing and OB/GYN, and I set out on this trail. My parents then had a personal tragedy. My only brother died at the age of 36. Afterwards, my parents couldn't handle running the hospital, so leadership was thrust upon me, and I took over the reins. I wanted to build a place where women could come to birth and feel safe. It started with that vision. To do that, I had to build a team.

Now, let's move forward. Within about 15 years, we became a referral center for complicated pregnancies, because word got around that there's a place with a team that works 24/7. It's protocol driven, so colleagues began to refer their mothers to us. That led to some very sick mothers being referred. Sadly, we couldn't save some of these young mothers because they just came too late. It tore me apart to see 22-year-old women dying on our watch. I began to read about maternal mortality and realized countries that reduced maternal deaths were countries that had invested in midwifery as a very strong workforce in maternal and newborn health services. India did not have anything like that.

I thought, "Let's approach the local government, the state where I work in, and ask if we could start midwifery training based on global standards." The government was not interested in anything that meant training beyond three months, so that's when I decided to pilot training in house. At the time, we were doing about 5,000 births a year, which meant we had enough volume to begin training. I had no idea how it was going to happen, what was going to happen, but we started the training.

We as obstetricians at Fernandez were considered to be a referral center, one of the best maternity services in the country. When I began to understand midwifery and read about it, it hit me. We were actually horribly interventional. The low-risk, healthy mother who came to us was caught in this crowd of complicated pregnancies, and she was also being treated as a catastrophe waiting to happen. If I had a mother who comes in labor, there is no need to start an IV line on her, but we were treating a variety of complicated pregnancies that we thought, "Uh oh. What if she bleeds? What if this happens? Let's not wait for that to happen. Let's start an IV line." That's ridiculous intervention that's not necessary. Somewhere along the line, we had lost focus, and when I realized that, I thought, "No. This is not right. We have built a place where mothers should feel safe, but we've lost focus and we're betraying the trust of mothers who come to us." That's when we decided we needed to change our childbirth practices.

That was a very important moment for me. I was probably two decades into my career, riding the crest and believing that I was a good obstetrician. I guess I was a good doctor in terms of skill and my love for my work, and I made sure I treated pregnancy as a natural event. When it came to the birthing room, we were interventional. That's what we had to change. That was the beginning of a very radical change, and we changed 180 degrees.

I realized then that I was drawn to midwifery. I was convinced that India needed midwives, not just to reduce maternal mortality, but also to reduce unnecessary cesareans, because at hospitals both private and public, cesarean section rates were as high as 75 percent, which meant out of every 100 women, only 25 were birthing normally. That was horrendous. I knew we had to train enough midwives to global standards and offer care to women, empowering them with knowledge, supporting them, and then straightaway see normal births start increasing and c-sections start decreasing.

I felt a tremendous calling to devote the rest of my professional life to promoting midwifery, to be an advocate for midwifery. Where are we today? Our purpose is to make pregnancy, labor, and birth safe for every pregnant woman walking through the doors of our hospitals. That is the purpose of Fernandez Hospital. Our job is to make sure that a pregnant woman, whether she's healthy or she's a woman with medical complications, has a journey to motherhood that is as safe as we possibly can make it.

How do we do this? We apply a collaborative model of care in which the primary carer will be the midwife, and wherever a woman needs more specialized inputs, then the obstetrician works along with the midwives. When we need more specialists like an endocrinologist if the mother has diabetes, then he or she comes into the picture. That is who we are today.

The midwife is really managing the case, but sadly, we don't have enough midwives to take care of the volumes that come to Fernandez. In October 2021, we oversaw births with 1,000 mothers. In November, it was a little more than 1,000. That's a very high volume for us. We don't have enough midwives to offer that one-on-one care for mothers. We need more midwives. Training is long and our standards are high.

It's a new profession being introduced in India. We're trying to motivate nurses to look at midwifery as career growth. The government made a commitment in December 2018 to introduce midwifery as a charter across the country. We're struggling at the moment. Our vision for India is that every pregnant woman is able to access midwifery care and to see an obstetrician only if required. At Fernandez, we believe if a low-risk healthy mother is being cared for by an obstetrician and if she is birthed by an obstetrician, then it's suboptimum care. We're trying to establish a very simple fact that women with no complications do not need obstetricians. They're far safer. Their birth experiences are more positive. **Outcomes are better in the hands of midwives.**

In one sense, having an obstetrician promote midwifery is a bit of a paradox in this country, because paychecks are linked with the number of births an obstetrician does. In Fernandez, we are very sheltered. We are privileged because all of us are on salaries. Nobody is being paid a fee for service. In the world outside, obstetricians are paid for every birth they are involved in. That's a huge challenge.

There's a lot of pushback from my fraternity. We've been in midwifery care now for the last 11 years. There are 4,000 private hospitals across the twin cities of Hyderabad and Secunderabad, and no other private hospital has introduced midwifery. That should show you the challenges we're working with. When our organization was asked by the state government to train nurses in midwifery, we grabbed it with both hands, because India has an annual birth rate of 26 million; 50 percent happens in private hospitals and 50 percent in public hospitals. They said, "Let's work in public hospitals because we are dealing with women from the lowest socio-economic group, and birth is a basic human right. If we can bring about change for the poorest woman in the state where I live, then our efforts are worthwhile."

We trained the first cohort in 2017, and the training was completed in 2019. Today, those 30 nurses call themselves agents of change. They are posted in clusters of three or more in district hospitals across the state, which are in small towns out at least anywhere between 3 hours or 6 hours from the capital, Hyderabad, where I live. Some of the hospitals are towards the edge of the tribal belt. These qualified midwives are doing amazing work. They have ensured that every woman has a birth companion. They have brought gym balls and the Rebozo into public hospital birthing rooms. They have created a sense of privacy with curtains. They encourage women to birth in the positions of their choice. They make sure there's skin to skin immediate breastfeeding, and they've reduced c-sections.

I can look into the eyes of any person and say, "The care being given in our public hospitals to the poorest woman is the same as in Fernandez Hospital to the people who pay for their care." I think that's what equitable health is all about.

The government of the state has absorbed this and has decided to create a unique task force. We've got a commitment of training 1,500 nurses for the state over the next four years. In other words, it is spreading, and the idea is to infiltrate all public hospitals across the state with midwives.

Now, how does it spread beyond the state of Telangana? Thankfully, The Ministry of Health and Family Welfare (MoHFW), Government of India sent a small group to verify the impact of midwifery care. The delegation spoke to the trainee midwives, mothers who received midwifery care and obstetric colleagues. This led to the Government's decision to establish midwifery-led care units across India's public hospitals.

Fernandez is recognized as a national training institute for midwifery educators. That's a whole different training program. Now, you need to remember we don't have midwifery in India, so we naturally do not have trainers to train the trainers. We advertised on social media and other places wherever we could enroll midwives from outside India. We've had midwives with clinical credibility and a passion for teaching from UK, Estonia, Denmark and Italy. Soon we will have midwifery trainers from New Zealand and the United States. The international midwives and qualified midwives of Fernandez together work alongside with the Trainees in both Fernandez and in the public hospitals of our state, preparing them to become future educators in midwifery.

We work with global agencies like UNICEF. UNICEF facilitated the training of midwives in our own state. WHO is helping us train nurses to become national midwifery educators. So, while these global agencies fund the bulk of the cost, we supplement the rest. The Fernandez Foundation not only offers technical help, but also provides a certain level of financial help. We believe it's worth it.

What we are trying to do is discover or look out for obstetric champions in the states where these future midwifery educators go back to work, and we're also trying to sensitize obstetricians and all levels of staff involved in birthing rooms to tell them what midwives do, why are they important, and what their role is in this plan from the government. Respectful maternity care is high on the government's radar and midwifery philosophy ensures midwives offer it to every woman in labour.

When you have 40 births in 24 hours, you don't have running water, beds, disposables, hospital sheets, or clothes for the patients to wear, how do you offer respectful care? The staff is not trained. They're trying to cope. There are also levels of corruption. When women walk into a public hospital, they're not supposed to pay for anything, but the staff is corrupt, so the woman ends up paying at different levels. We label this as "out of pocket" expenditure.

Now we are bringing midwifery into this atmosphere, and we are trying to instill a whole set of values. While the midwives are trying to implement respectful care, you've got other challenges. Nobody wants to talk about the elephant in the room, i.e., "out of pocket" expenditure via cash payments made to various levels of healthcare workers. The loss of this "pocket money" could result in moderate to severe "pushback" for midwifery care in public hospitals.

In a public hospital, where many births are taking place and they don't have enough staff, a cleaning lady (also known as a daya) who's been there for many years is fairly confident with helping that woman birth. The mother is grateful there is someone who has helped her birth. The daya who is not a nurse or a doctor, but staff in that room, cuts the cord and takes the baby away. The helpless mother then has to pay this woman to have her baby back with her.

These are horrendous stories. Often there are no covering sheets for the women in labour. So the staff will use the woman's sari to cover her, and she could be lying there in her urine and her feces for a fairly long time. People may not come to help her unless the woman pays for that help. In this kind of atmosphere, the midwives become lanterns of hope by offering compassionate, respectful, competent care.

We have visited the sites where the first cohorts of qualified midwives are posted in clusters in District hospitals. The ripples of change brought about by the midwives have permeated to the other staff in the birthing rooms. Because I was very moved when the cleaning staff and the housekeeping staff came up to me and said, "We don't know what you've done, but we know that you've done something very different because this nurse who worked here before has come back and is teaching us so many things. We are enjoying working again." There was a palpable sense of pride and joy in seeing an increase of normal births and a decrease in their need to refer mothers elsewhere. So I don't want to give up on what we are doing.

I think if globally all countries could absorb established midwifery as the backbone of their maternity services, we would reduce a lot of mental health issues, like postpartum depression and suicide among mothers. We would have happier, healthy mothers and healthy babies. Then you're involved in, as Julie says, "Birthing The New Humanity." Then you see the next generation that's not just being born but surviving and thriving. When you empower women during their pregnancy and give them the right advice on how to prepare to bond with their babies emotionally and psychologically and then you have a midwife supporting her, she will definitely have a positive birth experience. She then steps into motherhood on a very positive note. My God, can we ask for anything better than that?

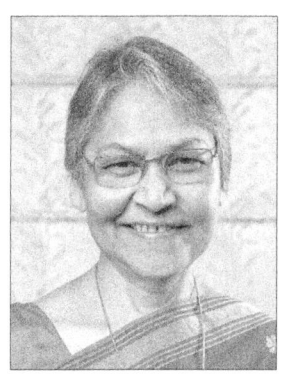 **Dr. Evita Fernandez** (FRCOG) is a renowned obstetrician and the chairperson of Fernandez Foundation, Hyderabad. She is a Fellow of the Royal College of Obstetricians and Gynaecologists, London. She strongly believes in the need to empower women to make choices, especially regarding issues surrounding birth. Dr. Evita is a champion of natural birthing and midwifery in India. She has spearheaded the country's first Professional Midwifery Education and Training (PMET) Programme. Her **PRO**fessional **MI**dwifery **SE**rvices (PROMISE) campaign is committed to creating a national cadre of professional midwives who are vital to the care of low-risk pregnant women. In a career spanning three decades, Dr. Evita has been at the forefront of maternal and newborn care in India.

Chapter 22

HUMANISING CHILDBIRTH

By Lesley Page, PhD

I qualified as a midwife in 1966. Since then, I've been a midwife in a number of roles. During that time of qualifying as a midwife in the sixties, there were two different forms of maternity care happening in the United Kingdom. There was community based and hospital care. I became a midwife in Scotland. We were already beginning a kind of factory approach to birth; we were trying to get more women into hospital, but we also had midwifery 'on the district' or in the community.

For half of my midwifery education, I was in the hospital. It was definitely a factory system. Women came into hospital in labour. As pupil midwives, we were called to the birth by a flashing light in the corridor. We might be working on the antenatal ward or the postnatal ward or the clinic, but when we saw this flashing light, we would rush up to the labour ward, racing other pupil midwives and medical students, and run into the woman's room to 'catch the baby'. We had to get 20 'deliveries', as they called them. We had to compete with medical students and midwifery students to get the 'delivery'. That's what we called birth.

We didn't get to know each woman ahead of time. We were there for the last minutes of the labour and for a few minutes after birth. The care was really fragmented. Women were cared for in the community and came to clinic in the hospital, and we would often do a whole row of abdominal palpations, just going along the row learning our abdominal palpation skills. Then, in the postnatal ward, women were separated from their babies. The babies were put into a nursery, and they were wheeled out every four hours for women to breastfeed. Breastfeeding was very common at that time. Then, the babies were taken back to the nursery, and we kind of sterilized the babies. We washed them in Phisohex, an antiseptic, which was later discovered to create brain damage when it was used in large quantities.

For some of the time, I was on the district, and I lived in a house with two qualified midwives—they were called sisters—and another pupil midwife. In the district around us, we attended women in their own homes and attended home births, and then we visited women at home afterwards in the postnatal period. This experience gave me a very, very different vision of birth. I was aware of the peace and the tranquility of home birth, whereas in the hospital it was all sort of adrenaline fuelled. Even at home, birth was becoming medicalized. Women didn't get out of bed in labour if the midwife was there. They stayed in their bed to give birth.

I have a vivid memory of being in a lovely room in a small house in Edinburgh with a bedside lamp lit. I remember a soft glow of pink. The baby arrived, and a few minutes later, the brothers and sisters ran into the room and jumped onto the bed to meet their baby sister. That vivid impression has stayed with me for my entire life.

I became a midwife after I qualified as a nurse. At that time, many went on to become midwives after qualifying as nurses. After I qualified as a midwife, I went back to nursing for a while. Partly because I loved the one-to-one relationships that I developed with patients. I was an intensive care nurse.

Then my husband, who was a family doctor, our two children and I emigrated to the north of Canada, and then eventually moved to Vancouver, British Columbia, Canada. An obstetrician that I had gotten to know through meeting at conferences asked if I would help set up the first legally recognized midwifery service in Canada.

At that time in Canada, women could only get midwifery care if they went outside of the system. Midwifery had no place in established health services, and it was seen as an alternative, even illegal. Bernd Wittman, my obstetrician friend, was keen to establish midwifery as a part of the health services in Canada.

I worked with three other "nurses" (we weren't allowed to call ourselves midwives) who had been qualified as "midwives"; one in the USA and three of us in the United Kingdom, and four obstetricians who wanted to see midwifery developed in Canada. In this practice project, we automatically provided continuity of care. We four midwives had a small caseload of women. This was in addition to our full-time jobs as educators in maternity nursing or perinatal nursing. In the practice, we provided all care—the antenatal care, care during labour and birth, care after birth—for a small group of women. As we got to know each other, women and midwives, the women would ask us questions. For example, at that time, women weren't allowed to eat or drink at all during labour. One woman asked me, "Well, why is that?" I couldn't answer her. I started to research the question.

I knew that some midwives in the Bronx in the USA had done some research. When I contacted them, they gave me the references and explained what they had learned. The reason women weren't allowed to eat or drink during labour was said to be because of possible Mendelson syndrome, aspiration of stomach contents during anaesthesia for caesarean section. We found that the evidence did not support restriction of fluids and food in labour. Because it was so important to women to be fed and hydrated, we got the policy changed.

Often, when we questioned a policy, it changed for the whole hospital. All sorts of other questions arose. Why were women kept in bed? Why couldn't they get up and move around? Why couldn't they squat? Why did we do episiotomies? About 90 percent of women had episiotomies, which is a cut in the perineum, the tissue between the vagina and the rectum or back passage. We started then to change many of our practices because of getting to know and listening to women.

But what was important to me was that I was part of the women's movement in Canada in the 1970s, when women were asserting the need for autonomy and playing their full role in the world. It seemed to me that women should have personal autonomy around the birth of their babies. This midwifery that we were practicing became focused on helping women retain personal autonomy and to choose the kind of birth that they wanted, as well as giving family-centered care, care focused on the needs of the woman, her baby and family.

I became absolutely captivated. We were getting to know women and their families intimately. We were there at the birth of their baby, the start of a new life, and the woman becoming a mother. She was being born as mother, and the family was coming together around this new baby. It just felt as though I was at the center of the world, being with women and their families at that special time.

We collected data about what was happening in our practice pilot and obtained the views of the women receiving care. The cesarean section rate in our practice was very low. The outcomes were good. Women were highly satisfied and were choosing to come to us. It became a model that helped establish midwifery as a legal profession with registration and regulation of midwives in British Columbia, Canada. This experience gave me a vision of how birth might be, and an understanding of the vital role midwives play.

I was eventually recruited to return home to the United Kingdom. I came to Oxford, where I still live today. I was appointed to be Director of Midwifery of a large maternity service for Oxford. In the United Kingdom, all women have midwifery care. Midwives work within the National Health Service looking after women during pregnancy, labour and birth and the period after birth. Oxford is a county that had two hospitals and community services, including home births and four small community hospitals. They were called cottage hospitals at the time. In total, there were 7,500 to 8,000 births a year. There were hundreds of midwives since midwives in the UK provide most of the care and are professionally autonomous.

Care had become very fragmented and was starting to be medicalized. When I returned from Canada, I could see that because of this, the role of midwifery had becoming more restricted and limited.

One of my ambitions in Oxford was to develop what we call continuity of carer—to go back to having midwives care for women through the whole process of pregnancy, labour, and birth and the early weeks of life. We set up a small team of midwives, so the women had their own midwife who provided most of the care but working in a small group practice so that women and midwives could get to know each other over time, developing a relationship of trust. Early research had been undertaken by Caroline Flint, called Know Your Midwife. From my work in Canada, I understood the power of the woman and her midwife having a relationship—getting to know and learning to trust each other over time. A relationship in which they could talk through the shorthand language of friendship.

We were featured in a BBC series called, "Your Life in the Hands," on primetime television. Around the world in many parts of the world, interest in continuity of care grew. Interest in the organisation that allows women and midwives to get to know each other over time.

I then went on to become the first professor of midwifery in the United Kingdom and was attached to Queen Charlotte's and

Hammersmith Hospitals in London, a National Health Service Trust. My first work as a professor was to lead in setting up a large-scale project called One to One Midwifery. For a large proportion of the women in that National Health Service Trust, over 5,000 women, about a fifth of them would be cared for by a named midwife who provided most of the care working in a small group of midwives—between six to eight midwives—providing continuity so that the woman was cared for during most of her pregnancy, labour, and birth, and after birth by a midwife and midwives that she knew.

We undertook a rigorous evaluation of clinical outcomes, of quality of care, of use of economic resources, and of the experience of women and of midwives. There was a higher normal birth rate. The care was safe. The outcomes for the baby were as good as they were with standard care. In other words, it was safe for the baby. Women had a very positive experience, and the midwives who wanted to work in that way also had a very positive experience. They said that they felt like real midwives for the first time. Economically, it cost no more and probably even cost less than the standard fragmented care.

Relationship-based care has been the theme of my work for much of my career. I was involved in the Department of Health expert maternity group, which wrote the policy Changing Childbirth. This changed the direction of maternity policy for England. Changing Childbirth was about woman-centered care; care that focused on the needs of women, rather than the needs of the Institution, giving women power to make their decisions about their own care. It marked a profound power shift. The woman, who chaired this expert group, Baroness Cumberlege, sits in the House of Lords, and is still leading the development of progressive policy for the National Health Service in England.

Continuity of carer is a vital part of what we call humanized childbirth. Midwifery Continuity of Carer has been established and evaluated in a number of high-income countries. It is usually led by midwives, but often with obstetricians' and government support. High quality randomised trials of midwifery continuity of care from around the world have been synthesised in the Cochrane Library. From the review of these trials conducted in many different countries, it is concluded that midwifery continuity of carer is associated with a lower preterm birth rate, a lower fetal loss rate, a higher vaginal or normal birth rate, lower interventions, and high satisfaction among women.

So from this high-quality evidence, we have an indication that this relationship-based care, working through a relationship with a woman and her family, has powerful consequences, leads to better health and experience. Based on current policy planning, continuity of care should be available to most women in England over the next few years, and similarly, in the three other countries of the United Kingdom.

In 2012, I was elected as President of the Royal College of Midwives. The Royal College of Midwives had at that time about 41,000 members, the majority of midwives in the United Kingdom. As President, I took every opportunity to travel around the United Kingdom and many other parts of the world, meeting midwives, doctors, women, their partners, their babies, doulas, and people working in the maternity services. I began to see progress being made in some parts of the world, but that there were real problems everywhere. However, there was hope! Childbirth was being reformed and humanized, and some were introducing midwifery continuity of carer, but often this reform was patchy.

Many mainstream services were fragmented and sometimes disrespectful, even abusive. In many parts of Europe and South America, for example, I learned about the Kristeller Maneuver, in which the doctor pushes on the woman's abdomen to push the baby out during labour. It's very dangerous, very painful to the woman, and dehumanizing. I learned about women being forced to stay in bed in stirrups, not having any choices, having enforced episiotomies, being treated disrespectfully, their wishes not being observed, having no control over the birth of their baby, and being treated cruelly. This is much more prevalent than we realise.

But at the same time, I realised that we had created a strong foundation for humanizing birth. Humanizing birth means supporting birth as a transformation, a transformation that gives the baby the best start in life and the woman the best start as a mother. A start that will set a foundation for long term health, wellbeing, happiness and strong relationships through life, and will impact on future generations. This contributes greatly to a better society.

Over time it occurred to me that the problems around childbirth that are associated with medicalisation, institutionalisation, and dehumanisation are as important as the climate crisis. They are as important as our destruction of the environment and come from the same roots—the belief that we can interfere in nature and can interfere in physiology to any extent without any costs. Of course, access to medical care is crucial, but the levels and rate of unnecessary intervention are high; high in much of the world, while some women have little or no access to high quality health care.

Humanizing childbirth has the potential to build on progress and resolve problems. It is a response to medicalisation, institutionalisation and dehumanisation. The aim must be to ensure access to high quality safe health care for every woman, her baby and family. Women need health services that will give the best possibility for health, wellbeing, happiness, positive mental health, delight and joy, as well as hope, around the birth of their babies. Of course, women must be able to choose when they become pregnant and if they want to give birth, but once they have made that choice, every woman, every baby in the world, and every family should have access to the care, which will give them the best start in life. Health and wellbeing are much broader concepts than, for example, reducing the stillbirth rate or reducing maternal mortality. These are essential goals, but we must move beyond the basic to consider how we can help each woman, her baby and family, have the kind of start that will meet their broader health, social, cultural and spiritual needs in the short and the long term.

We must see the world of childbirth in a different way. We need to see that our aim is not just survival; it's thriving. It's bringing about the best start in life, the start which will give this human being the opportunity to live well and contribute to a better world.

This will have an impact on all of us. Pregnancy, birth and early life is a critical, sensitive period. It is the only birth of this baby. A poor experience and poor care cannot be replaced. We can compensate, but we can never replace that experience, that birth of that baby. Ongoing health and the wellbeing of the woman, who has the right to optimal health and who needs to be healthy to look after her baby, the support for the relationship between mother, baby, and the other parent and family, create a foundation for long-term health, into old age, and ongoing loving relationships. This love between the mother and the baby is the first love relationship of that baby's life. Supporting rather than disturbing loving relationships and contributing to care that supports secure attachments are vital to the future of the baby. This early experience forms a template for future relationships and emotional wellbeing.

Our work as midwives gives us a particular calling. In Iceland, midwives are called Mother of Light. This comes from the idea that the midwife is with the woman when she brings her baby into the light of the world, but also means enlightenment using the knowledge that we have to help light the way we care for women around the birth of their babies. I think that respect for midwifery and all of those who work in childbirth in the birthing community, doulas, activists, maternity voices, and groups of people that work on *Womb to Thrive* make a huge contribution to a better society.

In medicalizing childbirth, our society has reduced its meaning. Much of humanizing birth is about understanding the significance of birth. Somehow, we must draw attention to this issue. For example, I would like to have the United Nations talk about the importance of humanizing childbirth. Individuals in the World Health Organization (WHO) have expressed interest in the concept. Women are often undervalued in much of the world, so the meaning of birth has been minimized, but this is the birth of human beings, the next generation. It's about this miracle of a life coming into existence. It is absolutely miraculous, and yet it's an everyday miracle.

Now, many people say that the birth of the baby is the birth of the world. The birth of the baby is a road to love and peace around the world. Of course, scientifically we can't prove those things, but when we go beyond our very limited science to understand the impact, we see that the way we look after women as they give birth to their babies will make the world so much better.

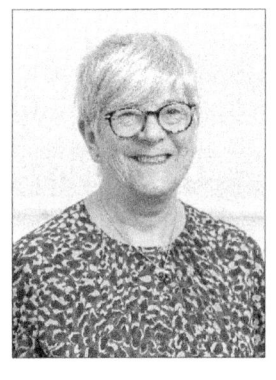 **Professor Lesley Page, CBE**, is a midwife living in the UK. Her career has spanned decades and many roles. She has been involved in hands-on practice, academic work, managing large services, and served as the President of the Royal College of Midwives in the UK for 5 years. She has developed national and international policy as well as international development of high-quality midwifery and maternity care. Her focus is on humanising childbirth, supporting the transformative power of pregnancy, birth, and the early weeks of life to give the best start in life and a better future.

Chapter 23

THE LIFE-ENHANCING SIGNIFICANCE OF A PHYSIOLOGICAL BIRTH

By Dr. Pooja Shenoy

I began my career as an obstetrician working with pregnant women and their families for 9 years. As an obstetrician, I was trained to look at birth as a medical event with frequent and unnecessary interventions in the birthing process. As much as I enjoyed working with mothers-to-be, I was unhappy with my professional life; something did not seem right. I also noted with increasing dismay the lack of respect, dignity, kindness, and compassion women in labour often suffered at the hands of my obstetric colleagues.

Their indifference towards pregnant women in their moments of vulnerability was difficult for me to fathom. Finally, I became a victim of obstetric violence myself, and then the picture got clearer; I realised that I could not continue working as an obstetrician. In 2017, with support from the Fernandez Foundation, I re-trained and became a doula and a birth educator.

A physiological birth is a birth that is devoid of any human intervention. The process is driven by a woman's innate ability to birth her baby at her own pace. Here, birth hormones orchestrate the event, as designed by evolution. Labour starts on its own and progresses without any time constraint. In such births, women have:

- the flexibility to enjoy uninterrupted movement
- the freedom to adopt positions of comfort
- the freedom to have food and fluids of their choice
- access to comfort measures they prefer and
- the ability to use natural expulsive reflexes to birth in positions of their choice.

When mothers birth babies normally, the mother-baby dyad remains undisturbed. The mothers can offer skin-to-skin care and start breastfeeding within the first hour of birth. The process ends with delayed cord clamping and allows mothers to birth the placenta spontaneously.

The normal physiology of childbirth remains intact when we allow births to progress without any interference. This empowers women and lets them own their birth experience. It also helps ensure that babies come into the world in a calm and gentle manner. They have a smoother transition to life outside the womb. These factors lead to better physical and emotional health in mothers and babies.

What's wrong with birthing today?

The birthing process is seeing widespread medicalisation, which has led women to stop trusting their own bodies. Women today have an acquired fear of childbirth due to:

- misconceptions in society,
- birth experiences often insensitively shared by family and friends, and
- a melodramatic picture portrayed through media

The medicalised environment in birthing rooms do nothing to ease their fears. With this on their minds, women go into labour thinking that the birthing process can only be managed medically.

Healthy birth practices

Instead of a medicalised approach to birthing, there is strong evidence for natural birthing practices that combine movement, posture, and diet.

Letting labour begin on its own is the best way to know that a woman's body is ready to go through labour and that the baby is ready to be born. In such births, gravity aids women when they move around and change positions. Movement and mobility help them stay active and in control of their bodies. Using movement and mobility is also the most effective way to distract their minds from the discomfort of labour. Often the positions and movements that bring comfort will also help labour progress. It is important to allow women to follow their instincts during labour to decide what works best for them. Research shows that movement and mobility reduce the duration of labour by up to one to one and a half hours, decreases the caesarean rate by 30 percent, and reduces the need for an epidural by 20 percent. The WHO 2018 recommendations on the intrapartum care for a positive childbirth experience also encourages the adoption of movement and mobility and an upright position during labour in women at low risk.

A woman who follows her body's natural instincts may find herself birthing in a gravity-assisted position. Some of these postures include:

- standing
- squatting
- side-lying or
- on all fours.

These positions are beneficial, as they help open the pelvis and use gravity to help the baby descend.

Diet is also important. Giving women in labour the freedom to eat and drink keeps their energy levels up and help them cope better with the increasing demands of labour. A 2017 systematic review of ten trials including nearly 4000 women found no evidence to support restrictions on what a woman should eat or drink in a typical labour.[1] If anything, restrictions may mean prolonged and more painful labour.

A successful physiological birth sets the stage for a gentler postnatal experience for both mother and baby. It allows for the next set of natural practices that are critical for the mother-child bonding and the long-term development of the child. The first step towards achieving this is keeping mothers and babies together skin-to-skin and starting the first breastfeed within one hour after birth (golden hour of birth). Studies have shown that babies held skin-to-skin right after birth:

- have stable temperatures and blood sugars
- cry less
- breastfeed sooner, longer, and easier
- more stable breathing and heart rate patterns and
- have a smoother transition to the world outside.

The mother holding the baby soon after birth and during the first hour after birth can also help in better bonding between mother and child.[2]

The second step while mothers and babies enjoy uninterrupted skin-to-skin contact is to wait until the cord pulsations stop. Waiting until then allows blood carrying iron-rich haemoglobin from the placenta to reach the baby.[3] This helps to improve the iron stores for the first several months of life and decrease the risk of anaemia.[4]

Steps to achieve physiological birth

It is important that women build confidence in their bodies and the birthing process. The first step towards that state is to empower them to gain knowledge about childbirth and receive evidence-based information. This knowledge will help them identify the birth team who will help them have the physiological birth they deserve. Women can then have access to birth tools and non-pharmacological comfort measures to cope with labour. Such a personalised birth environment helps achieve an enriching and memorable birth experience.

Antenatal education is key to building a woman's confidence and overcoming her fears. The availability of adequate and proper information helps minimise the possibility of over-medicalisation. As a childbirth educator, I provide unbiased, evidence-based information to pregnant couples which helps them make informed decisions during pregnancy, labour, and childbirth. Through antenatal education, the pregnant woman learns to follow a healthy lifestyle through the course of her pregnancy to keep her body fit in preparation for labour and birth, and to understand how her mind, body and baby work together in synchrony during labour. Labour can be discomfiting and stressful, so the woman is taught coping strategies as a crucial means of support.

Some of these strategies can draw in a wider circle of support for the woman. Fernandez Hospital, for example, encourages support groups for pregnant women, offering a wider circle of support to her. Through pregnancy support groups, the woman can connect with her peers, receive evidence-based information and share birth experiences, which further empowers her on this journey. Such groups are indeed a great bridge to a healthy parenthood.

The birth companion plays a key part of the birth team. This person is encouraged to attend antenatal education classes along with the mother-to-be, in which he/she is taught simple tools and techniques that would help him/her provide physical and emotional support to the woman during labour. I have noticed that, when birth companions attend the antenatal education classes, they feel more involved and empowered to provide meaningful support during labour.

The woman's birth team is constituted by a loved one, an obstetrician and/or a midwife, an intrapartum nurse and/or a doula; with each individual playing a distinct role in a woman's journey to motherhood. A Cochrane systematic review in 2017 concluded that women who receive continuous support during labour and birth have shorter labours, increased rate of spontaneous vaginal births, decreased usage of intrapartum analgesia, reduced caesarean birth rates, and increased overall satisfaction with the birth experience.[5] Labour companionship has also been recommended as a part of the WHO 2018 intrapartum guidelines for a positive childbirth experience.

The role and the value added by each member of the birth team is outlined here:

- **Obstetrician:** The obstetrician is primarily responsible for the overall clinical and medical well-being of both mother and baby. This professional may not always be present during labour and will be caring for many other pregnant women along with clinical management, documentation, hospital policies, and other obligations. They provide care to pregnant women with complex needs and carry out interventions/surgeries if needed.
- **Midwife:** The midwife provides clinical care along with offering physical and emotional support to the woman in labour. She is trained to recognise deviations from the normal and escalate it to her obstetric colleagues. They then work collaboratively in providing the emergency care needed at that time.
- **Intrapartum nurse:** The intrapartum nurse offers clinical care as directed by the obstetrician or midwife in line with hospital practices. She is trained to provide support and comfort to the mother and to keep the obstetrician/midwife informed.

- **Husband/loved one:** The husband/loved one offers continuous support to the woman during labour. He/she is emotionally connected to the pregnant woman and offers varying amounts of comfort and support to the woman.
- **Birth Doula:** A doula is completely focused on offering continuous emotional support, physical comfort, non-clinical advice, and guidance for the mother.

Within my experience as a birth doula, I focus on offering physical, emotional, and informational support to the woman in labour. Physically, I help her with movement, mobility, and positioning, massages, and offering different techniques of relaxation and comfort measures, generally ensuring that her basic needs during labour are met. Emotionally I provide her with reassurance and encouragement as she goes through labour. I do not make decisions for her but provide her with evidence-based information so that she is empowered to make choices. I also provide support to the birth companion so that he/she can support the woman better in labour in ways that are comfortable to them. As a doula, I do not give medical advice or intervene clinically during labour.

At our workplace, towards term, we encourage every pregnant couple to write down and discuss their birth preferences with their birth team. Voicing and discussing birth preferences encourages effective communication with the birth team regarding choices and preferences during labour and childbirth to ensure the best possible experience and outcome. Birth preferences can include who the woman would want as her birth companion, her thoughts on movement and mobility, her attitude towards pain relief, her choice of comfort measures, and the birth environment she would like. (Dim lights, use of music, birth affirmations, fragrances and candles, etc.)

We also provide a variety of non-pharmacological comfort measures. These include the availability of food and fluids, hot and cold fomentation, visualization and visual focus, use of birth affirmations, warm showers and birth pools for hydrotherapy (water immersion for relaxation and pain relief), breathing techniques, music, aromatherapy, massage, and acupressure. All these comfort measures ensure that the woman in labour stays relaxed through the process, thus ensuring that the right hormone (oxytocin) production is maximised during labour. The WHO 2018 guidelines on intrapartum care for a positive childbirth experience also mention similar measures to which women in labour should have access to.

The objective is to create a quieter, calmer, gentler, and more soothing birth environment. When I was working as an obstetrician, I never realised how draining a highly medicalised environment could be for birthing women. The frightening array of medical equipment only aggravates the fears associated with the pain in labour. In my experience, I have seen that by just keeping the lights low, adjusting the room temperature as per the woman's preference, playing some calm music, offering birth affirmations, and adding fragrances that promote relaxation go a long way in keeping a birthing mother relaxed and in control of her labour.

We also provide a variety of birth tools like birth balls, peanut balls, rebozo, CUB, birth stools, and massage tools that not only support physiological birth but also enhance movement, comfort, and adoption of positions. With the availability of these simple cost-effective and useful birth tools, I see women navigating easily and instinctively through their labour and having positive birth experiences. The Royal College of Midwives (RCM) states that the help of simple birth tools like birth balls, chairs, and rebozo, more women can enjoy the benefits of a physiological birth.[6]

It is important that every woman builds up confidence in her body and the birthing process. For this to happen at the community level and the world at large, it is vital that the professionals involved in the care of pregnant women understand the physiology of birth and how hormones orchestrate the birthing process. Secondly, pregnant women today are often victims of disrespectful care and obstetric violence. This leads to birth trauma and post-traumatic stress disorder. Medical school curriculum should include sensitisation in respectful maternity care. Thirdly, care-providers working with pregnant women should receive adequate training to build their own confidence to support women who wish to have physiological births. Finally, obstetricians should understand the value a professional midwife brings to pregnancy, birth, and postpartum experience.

As most pregnant women have uncomplicated pregnancies, they can be cared for only by a midwife. Obstetricians can then focus on the minority of pregnant women who have complicated pregnancies, and even in this subgroup, women can benefit from midwifery support. This way we can ensure that many pregnant women benefit from the collaborative care of both an obstetrician and a midwife.

Data available shows that over half a million women worldwide die of pregnancy-related complications each year and a still larger number of infants suffer the same fate. Midwifery care would go a long way in reducing this horrifying statistic, particularly in areas where access and availability of obstetric care is limited, as is the case in most underdeveloped/developing countries.

We need to understand that every birth will unfold with its own uniqueness. With a little help from birth professionals, every woman has the power to make birth a positive experience and emerge as a stronger and more confident individual.

References
1. Ciardulli, Andrea, et al. "Less-restrictive food intake during labor in low-risk singleton pregnancies." Obstetrics & Gynecology 129.3 (2017): 473-480.

2. Moore ER, Bergman N, Anderson GC, Medley N. Early skin-to-skin contact for mothers and their healthy newborn infants. Cochrane Database of Systematic Reviews 2016, Issue 11. Art. No.: CD003519. DOI: 10.1002/14651858.CD003519.pub4
3. McDonald, Susan J., et al. "Effect of timing of umbilical cord clamping of term infants on maternal and neonatal outcomes." Evidence-Based Child Health: A Cochrane Review Journal 9.2 (2014): 303-397.
4. American College of Nurse Midwives. "Delayed umbilical cord clamping." (2014).
5. Bohren, Meghan A., et al. "Continuous support for women during childbirth." Cochrane Database of Systematic Reviews 7 (2017).
6. Jenkinson, Bec, Natalie Josey, and Sue Kruske. "BirthSpace: An evidence-based guide to birth environment design." (2014).

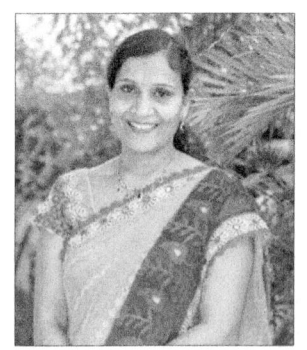

Dr. Pooja Shenoy is a Lamaze-certified childbirth educator, a certified birth doula, a certified hypnobirthing practitioner, a BPNI-certified lactation counsellor, and an infant massage practitioner at the Fernandez Foundation. She empowers pregnant women to overcome their fears of childbirth and provide them with evidence-based information to help them make informed decisions. She continues to support women through labour, thus helping them have a positive birth experience.

Chapter 24

CHANGING THE WORLD, ONE BIRTH AT A TIME

By Anthea Thomas

It never occurred to me as I was growing up that the transformation into womanhood, the experience of childbirth, and becoming a mother were sacred life events that would change me so deeply.

After many years of life experience and deep personal growth, I began to reflect on how I experienced these rites of passage and saw the lost opportunity that I (and so many) face from the myths and misunderstandings passed down through the ages that have sadly become ingrained as our cultural norm.

Western culture particularly seems to exhibit a widespread disconnect from the foresight of other cultures, the significance of celebrations and support, but most importantly the trust in the immense power of our innate wisdom (mind and body).

As a society, we have lost our way in focusing on what is most important. Birth has become a medical event (1 in 3 women worldwide report their births as traumatic), and rates of medical intervention have increased consistently over the last 20 years.

As science has supposedly advanced, this disconnect has become more obvious as our physical and emotional health has continued to decline. We seem to trust more in pharmaceuticals and medical establishments than our incredible bodies that are far more advanced than any science could be.

I am grateful that my own journey has led me to where I am planted now, helping to change our birth culture so these seasons of life can be positive and experienced without fear and trauma. I found a deep passion for not only being a strong advocate for women but also working in a field in which I can support and share knowledge to help others find their inner strength and trust in their natural abilities.

Looking back, I remember feeling quite awkward as I blossomed from an adolescent girl into a young woman growing up in Australia. I did all I could to hide the many changes in my body and any evidence of my body bleeding in those first years. I know that many of my friends had similar experiences. Childbirth wasn't something we spoke about often, but when it was discussed, it sounded scary and incredibly painful, and we perceived it as a trauma that all women must face to become a mother. I pushed those beliefs and fears deep down into my sub-conscious, as it seemed to me like a faraway concept.

Life tends to have a habit of sneaking up on us, and before I knew it, my life had fast forwarded, and I was married and pregnant. These fears I had ignored were now right in front of me, and I was overcome with the prospect of facing them. I was excited about bringing a new life into our world, but my fear was intense, and I did anything to distract myself from the reality I faced.

We attended the hospital childbirth classes (which increased my fears), and we were shown ways to overcome the pain and negative experience by all the available interventions and narcotics. Here was my get-out-of-experiencing-birth card. I had mentally checked off all the options offered on this list, not knowing (or being told) how any of these medical interventions could affect my baby.

I could share many pages with you on the intimate details of my births, but I'm going to give you a much shorter snapshot of the tragedy that unfolded.

At 39 weeks of pregnancy (while still not facing my fears), labour began spontaneously, but soon I had a massive placental abruption, and our precious baby girl, Mackenzie, was cut off from her life support and was stillborn many hours later. We were absolutely devastated, and everything I had believed about birth came true, yet it was even worse than I had first imagined. With empty arms, we came home completely broken.

Losing a child and the grief that we held is hard to explain, but some very dark days followed and infiltrated every part of who we both were.

After doing all I could to avoid birth, I began to want it more than anything. We were blessed to find out we were pregnant almost 6 months after the birth and loss of our precious little girl.

This next pregnancy, even though it was all I wanted, was shrouded in even more fear, and we looked to our obstetrician to lead the way so that our baby would be safe. I had wanted to have another natural birth, but at 37 weeks, my obstetrician felt that an induction would be best due to my increasing anxiety. My body and my baby were not ready, and what followed was the cascade of unnecessary interventions. As the chemicals in my body were increased, labour became almost unbearable, and I was in full fight-and-flight mode. After 9 hours of artificial surging, our baby became distressed, and we ended up having an emergency c-section for which I was completely unconscious and not even aware of my daughter's birth.

We held our beautiful baby girl, Matilda, in our arms. I was grateful but traumatized by this violent experience of birth. Birth was not positive, and it would be many years before I could contemplate having another child and facing the prospect of the trauma that was childbirth.

In the 5 years between Matilda's birth and becoming pregnant again, I suffered from this trauma, and it impacted every part of who I was. I had no trust in myself and in my body, and I felt like a failure. I now know that this an all-too-common experience after a traumatic or disappointing birth, but at the time, I felt very alone.

I knew that I needed support with this new pregnancy. I wanted to have a more positive birth, but I had no idea who I could turn to. A friend suggested HypnoBirthing classes, but the name really put me off straight away. It sounded very alternative (a bit hippy), and I had visions of a hypnotist burning incense while I birthed in an eerie trance to their swinging pendulum and creepy chanting. It didn't sound like something that I aligned with at all.

I started researching our options, but all that I found was the hospital classes that I had already experienced in my previous pregnancies. So, with trepidation, I contacted the HypnoBirthing Educator to find out more. I was surprised that the classes were being run by a local midwife. She assured me that the course did not follow alternative methods but that it was a comprehensive antenatal course that was evidence based and supported by many midwives and obstetricians. That assurance got my attention, as I had grown up with a great respect for anyone in a white coat and medical degree! When I shared my story with her, she said that she had seen many couples experience phenomenal births after previous traumatic births, and HypnoBirthing could give me the trust in my body that I needed for my VBAC. I still had my doubts, but I had a lot of hope, so we booked her for 5 sessions.

This was the best decision and investment I think I have ever made! HypnoBirthing not only changed my pregnancy and birth, it also completely transformed my life!

Marie Mongan (the founder of HypnoBirthing) came across the work of Dr. Grantly Dick Read in the 1950s and used his theories to birth her babies in a calm and gentle manner, free of fear and the tension that creates pain (fear-tension-pain syndrome) that so many experience. I was impressed that this woman's vision for her own births had ended up impacting hundreds of thousands of women (couples) to confidently birth with this philosophy and these techniques. Little did I know that, at that time, Marie (Mickey) would become a close colleague, mentor, and friend to me, and her influence would change my path so greatly.

Over the next 5 weeks, we attended the classes, and I was immediately taken aback at how logical the information was. I was amazed to learn about my uterus that knew how to conceive, nurture, and birth my baby (all without my conscious control). I was shocked to learn about the history of birthing and why I and so many others have become so fearful of birth. When we explored the mind-body connection (neuroscience), and how integral it was to how we birth, the realization of why I had experienced such extreme fear and tension in my first two births became very evident.

My husband and I left the first class with a sense of relief and confidence. The fear we both held was already starting to melt away. We were highly motivated to apply all of our effort into practicing these techniques. We watched a birth video at the end of the first class that will be etched in my mind forever.

Hypnosis was the element of HypnoBirthing that I didn't feel comfortable with. It surprised me that hypnosis was not about someone controlling your mind, but a natural, relaxed state that we each experience every day, where we can access a part of our mind that is incredibly powerful and highly suggestible, so beliefs around birth (or anything) could be easily replaced and make way for a more positive outcome. Once I understood hypnosis, I looked forward to working with these mindset techniques and the possibility of changing my deep beliefs and fears.

Our birth partners play an integral role in birth, and I loved that the HypnoBirthing course not only focused on the birthing person, but also the members of the whole team. My supportive and loving husband, Paul, approached the classes with an open mind and enthusiasm. He was deeply affected by the loss of our daughter and felt helpless as our births unfolded into chaos. I could see immediately that he was benefiting from the information and keen to learn how to be a supportive advocate for this next birth.

We not only gained knowledge on the process of birth, the incredible hormonal flow and how to protect it, but we also absorbed a new birth mindset and confidence that was built in stages over the weeks that gave us an impenetrable belief in ourselves and our birth goals.

We learnt about pre and perinatal psychology (a field of study that has shown that babies are cognizant in the womb), shifted our focus from the physical experience of birth to understanding the importance of making informed decisions for whatever turn birthing took since the imprint of this time in the womb and birth is carried with them throughout life.

Through practicing the breathing techniques, daily guided relaxations, visualisations, affirmations and mind/body preparations, our fears continued to melt away. The biggest shift was after experiencing a powerful 'fear release with hypnosis', where we were supported to mentally release any fears, limiting beliefs and experiences that could hold us back from having the birth we wanted. Many of our fears are likely to show up during the birth if we haven't dealt with them, so it was important to face these head on, and allow them to be replaced in the subconscious. It is such a simple process, yet so powerful. Following this release, I felt like a dark cloud had lifted, and a sense of complete trust and power was unleashed.

I had struggled initially to relax down in hypnosis, but with daily practice, I found myself able to reach a deep state of relaxation almost instantly, and it surprised me, as I was someone who generally had a busy mind, and relaxation did not usually come easily. Our excitement grew and by 40 weeks of pregnancy, we couldn't wait for labour to begin.

The pressure was mounting (as my OB became nervous), but we worked together with him day by day to ensure our baby was safe, and finally our little boy was ready at 42 weeks!

It really isn't important how this birth played out (although, it was truly incredible). This birth enabled me to find my true inner power! The process of finding my inner confidence and experiencing this 'rite of passage' and using the wisdom of my body and mind, so that my baby could have a gentle and positive birth, was incredible! I did it!!

This birth healed me in so many ways, and I knew immediately that if I could transform from such intense fear to complete confidence, then this program would help so many others.

I believed so deeply in what I had learned that I left my corporate career and became trained as a HypnoBirthing Educator. I started teaching the program to pregnant couples. I was excited to see the impact the program was having on the families I worked with. I became a doula and began to witness the miracle of birth and the power that this education was having on so many.

I went on to study Hypnotherapy and Hypnofertility. In 2014, I stepped up to run the Australian division of HypnoBirthing International, providing training and support for new educators. In 2019, I was invited to become the VP of the HypnoBirthing Institute helping to steer the organization (46 countries) along a path to greater heights. It's been a phenomenal journey, and I am so grateful for it.

My story is unique to me, yet no more important than each of our stories and the path that it has led us to experience. I'm sure there are gifts and learnings (silver linings) in all we experience, and when we look for them, they are always there.

There is no failure in birth (or life), but there is a failure in the systems and culture of how we view and experience birth (and life). We have in front of us an opportunity (and responsibility) to change it for future generations by sharing our knowledge and insights. Each of us plays an important role in guiding the next generation, and our words and actions affect the way our children (and those in our influence) experience these sacred milestones in their life. Can you imagine the impact on future generations if we taught our daughters about their inner power and strength and show them the celebration and support they can feel as they approach these beautiful milestones?

HypnoBirthing International is now recognized as a world leader in providing premium childbirth education in more than 46 countries. The evidence-based program is taught by our educators and is helping to create safer, more comfortable, and more positive birth experiences. It has impacted hundreds of thousands of birthing families worldwide.

The HypnoBirthing philosophy and toolbox for birth and beyond supports all birth choices and prepares the birthing family for the best possible birth experience they can have. The core of this approach is not in how or where we birth (as birth can be unpredictable), but about how we feel. The HypnoBirthing course and tools help us tap into our inner strength and power, and when we do, we change the world, one birth at a time.

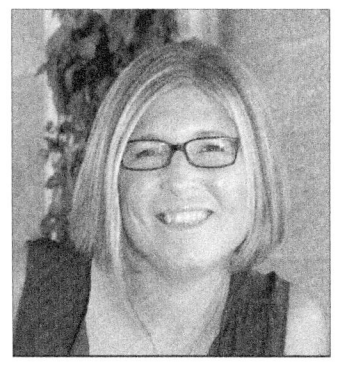

Anthea Thomas CH.t, HBCE, HBFC, is a passionate health professional, an experienced Ante-natal Educator, Doula, Speaker, and Hypnotherapist supporting families in conception, pregnancy, birthing, and parenting. Anthea is the Vice President of the HypnoBirthing® Institute. She is the Director of HypnoBirthing International in Australia, a Global Presence Ambassador for Parenting 2.0, and a member of the leadership team of CAPEA QLD (Childbirth and Parenting Educators of Australia).

http://www.hypnobirthing.com.au
(Australian website)

http://www.hypnobirthing.com
(Global website)

anthea@hypnobirthing.com.au
(Email)

Chapter 25

WHAT NEW PARENTS NEED TO KNOW

By Amélie Paterne

I lay in a hospital bed receiving my third blood transfusion. The medical staff were trying to save my life after I had just lost the one that had grown inside me. Far from my family and friends, I felt alone. My partner was by my side, but I knew somehow that he was not the right one for me. I felt so lonely and powerless. I even wondered what I had done wrong to end up in this situation. I was too weak for surgery, and life was draining from me. I remember a nurse tell me that I would forget this experience the day I held my future baby in my arms. This wasn't at all helpful. All I wanted to do was to leave London, return to France, and start a new life. Although it took me just over a month to recover physically, emotional recovery was another story. There was no emotional support for mothers who had faced miscarriages, as they were considered to be ordinary events.

I lost my job, and my whole life collapsed. Later, back in France, I realized that I had been in a toxic relationship, the pregnancy hadn't been planned, and I hadn't been ready to become a mother. *There was a reason behind all of this*, I thought. A few months later, I started a new job and a new life. I finally accepted the experience, but the fact that I had almost died made it more traumatic for me. Thanks to my spiritual teacher and my practice of Qigong, I worked on connecting with my inner resources and started to heal and be empowered. Even though my first pregnancy experience was quite the opposite of thriving, I am grateful for what it taught me.

Two years later, I first met my son's father. Although he wasn't sure he wanted another child, my intuition told me that a soul wanted to be born into our family. I could feel, deep down inside, that I was going to have a son. I remember the sensations through my whole body which brought me tears of joy. I got pregnant shortly afterward. My partner recognized how gifted we were to welcome this new life and give a brother to his 8-year-old daughter. This time, my environment was so much more stable and reassuring. My relationship was healthy, and we were very happy together. Although my first experience of pregnancy was far away, I could still feel the scar deeply imprinted in my cells and in my subconscious mind. This time, early in my pregnancy, I started to talk to my baby. I also wrote letters to him, telling him how I felt, what was going on in our lives, and how impatient his sister was to meet him.

Despite my first experience, I was now deeply convinced that I could trust my body through the birth process, so I looked for a midwife who taught hypnosis. I completed the birth preparation on my own, and I felt very confident, empowered, and close to my baby. I had a wonderful experience birthing my son using self-hypnosis techniques. The birth process, without an epidural or medication, lasted less than three hours. The midwives and doctors were amazed at how peacefully and comfortably I birthed my baby. Could it have been even better? Could I have received more support and information? The answer is definitely yes! I wish my son's father had been more involved and supportive during the birth and when we were back home.

As a young woman, I've always heard this beautiful sentence: **"becoming a parent will change your life forever"**. One can't fully comprehend the deep meaning of this sentence until actually becoming a parent, and many feel that they wish they had known more before they became parents." This personal experience changed me deeply, and I realized that, even if the birth was beautiful, I still wasn't fully prepared, and my partner was even less ready.

I knew I couldn't keep this knowledge to myself. In 2017, I became a HypnoBirthing – Mongan Method childbirth educator upon completing a training given by Julie and François Gerland. Since then, I have had the joy and the privilege of empowering other parents to experience a safer, easier, and more comfortable birth. I have become so passionate about helping future parents better prepare for parenthood, and I love making a difference in their lives. The classes I offer include teaching the critical importance of the prenatal period for the baby's development and how both mother and father can bond with their baby in utero. By doing this, they create a deep relationship based on unconditional love, care, and interaction. This becomes a way of life for the family, and the child then always feels that they are wanted and loved, belong, and can blossom in this world.

I also find it essential to teach couples to trust the mother's body through the birth process. I love seeing how individuals change when they connect with their inner guidance, emotions, and the body's intelligence. At the end of each class, they often say how ready they feel to birth their baby. I repeat the following to them and to myself: "Remember, no one is asking you to be a perfect mother or father. Just be present in the moment. If we had known better, we could have done things differently. Please be kind to yourself. We are all doing our best, and we all need reassurance." Parenting is such a responsibility and a vast undertaking. If parents received more holistic education and support before and after having children, so much suffering could be prevented.

The good news is that parents are increasingly willing to learn and do things differently. I meet many couples who want to be fully conscious and involved in the birth of their baby. However, they face many challenges. For example, the majority of women I work with have a professional life. Often, like men, their career gives them a sense of personal fulfillment they don't want to give up. Maternity leave here in France is a great start to enabling women to continue in their careers, but mothers can only take two months off from work, and fathers only receive a month. Mothers need more involvement from their partners in looking after the baby, as women don't envisage having a baby as their own project. They want both members of the couple to be fully engaged together.

Most of the mothers I teach say they don't have sufficient physical and emotional support to really blossom into their family and professional life.

This lack of support comes not only from the overworked health professionals who lack the time to focus beyond the physiological part of pregnancy, but it also involves the father. New dads are usually overwhelmed and don't really know how to help. This leads many women to lean on support from their friends. They may ask their mothers, mothers-in-law or grandmothers and search the internet for advice and information.

Women often experience high levels of fear, unknowing, self-doubt, and confusion as they try to navigate the different opinions they receive. The lack of good holistic education leads women to feel disconnected from their inner voice and natural instincts. Similar feelings arise when it's time to give birth. Most women expect the doctor or midwife to do the work, as they feel disconnected from their body and what's going on inside. They feel powerless and later express regret and pain regarding the whole process because it was out of their control. They wish they had been more informed and prepared to make choices for a more empowered birthing experience.

Importantly, fathers are increasingly willing to be more involved in the birth process. They just need to know they are wanted and needed and to be shown their place. This is how my role as a childbirth educator brings such important input.

Fortunately, HypnoBirthing, the Mongan Method, has pioneered the inclusion of fathers at the birth, offering them precise details regarding how they can support their partners and their babies. During these classes, the father or a birth companion chosen by the mother learns several techniques and methods to take an active role right from the beginning. If we want to thrive, everyone must play their part in creating stronger, more bonded, and more loving families.

Parenting is recognized as the hardest job in the world, yet there's no education on how to be a parent. Let's share the message that, along with professional diplomas, we must all receive education on how to become parents. When we think of our parents, we all probably agree that they would have done a better job if they had been well advised and supported. Of course, they did their best, but to create a thriving human family and planet, we must take parenting more seriously and be more prepared. We cannot just rely on cultural and medical habits, the popular and over-dramatised media mixed with confusing advice from family or close friends.

Albert Einstein said it so clearly when he wrote, "You can't fix the problem with the same mentality that created it." As well as healthcare workers, we need to teach youth, future parents, parents, and grandparents, as they all have an influence on young couples.

Future mothers and fathers have a natural instinct to bring new life into the world. They need to be empowered to ensure that they and their children will stop the current momentous trend of fear and trauma. Only then can they hope, as called upon in recent United Nations documents, to reach their full potential and thrive.

I believe that children can show us what we adults really seek. If they are not traumatized and are given fertile conditions to develop holistically, they help us reconnect within ourselves, thanks to their imagination, creativity, and spontaneity. They know how to be in the present moment, and these characteristics make them wonderful teachers. I tell couples that this is a mutual upliftment contract.

Parents should be aware that most of the souls who are willing to experiment life on Earth are probably older and wiser than them. My son, for example, was always older than his biological age. At just three years old, he told me that he came from the stars before arriving in my womb. I learn every day from him. My son is my masterpiece, my driving force, and he has helped me realize my life's mission. When we perceive parenting as a mutual exchange, it changes the way we relate and behave with each other.

Of course, everyone is free to choose their parenting style. I choose to live my daily life close to my son. It offers me the best playground and teaches me how to love and especially how to be in the present moment and accept emotions. We grow together, enjoying each other's company and life. You too can make this decision and choose this way to live. It is possible to be a fulfilled mother or father and to be a happy, healthy, thriving human being who follow their dreams, even big dreams, such as mine, to make a global impact.

I feel so grateful to live my passion, raise my son, and give him the best start in life so he too can live his full potential and create the life he wants feeling loved, supported and connected to his inner world and Mother Earth.

Becoming a parent doesn't mean that you should forget yourself and sacrifice your life, desires, needs, or dreams. On an airplane, parents are instructed to put their oxygen masks on first before helping their children. They have to look after themselves to have the strength to take care of their family.

Being a role model is probably the most important job for a parent, as children are imitators. If you treat yourself and others with kindness and respect, your children will follow your example. When I went to Brazil to help our group present on the importance of prenatal life at an international conference, I was away from my 3-year-old son for the first time. To my great surprise, his only comment on my return was, "I'm so proud of you, Mummy."

I have had the enriching experience of learning from and working with my mentors, François and Julie Gerland. Through their trainings and personal sessions to heal trauma and overcome my limitations, I am continually reaching new horizons. I have traveled with them as their Youth Delegation mentor to the World Family Organization Summits in Sao Paulo and Geneva, and I was even honored with an award for my work with the youth. I joined François and Julie on trips to a birth center in a slum and an international conference in India. These are just a few of the incredible experiences I have had as an integral part of their global family.

I recently began co-training professional HypnoBirthing childbirth educators with Julie and François. As a newly trained BirthTheChange® Facilitator and Director of BTNH World and through the Birthing The New Humanity App, we are able to spread our reach, inspire, inform and empower many more people across the globe.

My greatest wish for the world is for every young man and woman to feel empowered and ready to welcome a new life. Through harmonization between masculine and feminine principles, every human being can be born through conscious conception, feeling wanted and loved unconditionally, with parents empowered to recognise that they are conscious in the womb. During this time, mothers and fathers lay the foundations for lifelong health, wellbeing, creativity, and intelligence. This is outlined in the United Nations Framework for Early Childhood Development.

I deeply believe we all have the power to make the change we want to see in this world, and this starts in each of us and from the beginning of life. Today's situation is but a reflection and the consequences of our previous thoughts, desires and actions. Changing our perspective on the way we come to Earth will surely impact the future of humanity.

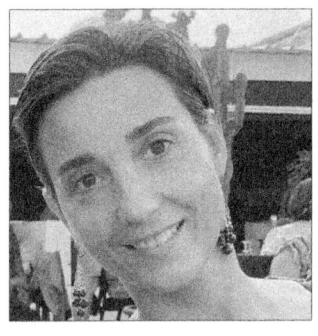 **Amélie Paterne** is a founding member and director of BTNH World Pte. Ltd. Their mission is to change early parenting and birth practices so every human being can thrive from the beginning. After giving birth naturally 9 years ago her passion to help couples live happy, comfortable pregnancies and births led her to teach HypnoBirthing: The Mongan Method. She currently co-trains educators and is actively launching the BTNH App with a global team of experts.

Chapter 26

NURTURE NATURALLY

By Effath Yasmin

The World belongs to those who dare to conquer it.

As a child, I felt I had no direction in life except for my burning belief in those words that rung in my heart. I struggled at school. My mom did the best that she could do in terms of trying to get me to cope with my schoolwork while most of my early years' teachers belittled and dismissed my efforts except for one who instilled a thought that I had a gift that needed an environment to blossom. That shifted during the crucial academic year of the tenth grade. I resolved to work harder and removed the few distractions I had and focused inward, which I later discovered is my *only* way to reflect and learn. It was my tryst with abyss of knowledge there is to discover in this lifetime. That desolated hopelessness turned into an unsatiable anticipation of what awaited me.

Without a doubt, that year was my defining moment in my life that revealed to me — my own light.

As I moved through high school, college and university, anything that came my way I was always willing to learn — almost like I had a fire in my belly, which I now consider is the greatest gift from God. It didn't really matter what was coming my way. All that mattered to me was what it had for me to learn. I came from an orthodox family background and culture and also a dysfunctional one at its core with no safe spaces to communicate without the risk to outrage a family member or to express oneself. We, as young girls and women of the household, were allowed very limited freedom. It was more the circumstances of family dysfunction or hardship that allowed me the most important opportunities from becoming financially independent or choosing my own life partner — Daniel.

Gaping wounds since childhood of sexual abuse, humiliation from not being good enough in the formative years at school, repressed anger watching my mother go about her choking life without a whimper all rolled into one. These defined my rebellious choices that I continued to make in an attempt to let my mother relive or liberate her lost life almost as if it were being weaved together to provide a *womb to thrive* for her. What I perhaps hadn't realized is how my choices could have given her more shattered glass to walk on. Yet the stoic silence she carried in her always spoke to my heart and gave me comfort that despite the sharp edges of my choices, she found her liberation through her progeny.

Fear and anger can be dismounting in life yet when we allow these emotions to flow instead of freeze us, it can become a pivotal force of change. It's almost as if these primal forces align with many other forces in the universe to become a catalyst that uplifts and changes your path. That feeling of surrender has reiterated itself many times later in my life.

Life after marriage ushered in a new beginning of doubtfulness or was it a new beginning of eventual possibilities? I was yet to find this truth. Sixteen years ago, I remember I was on the last round of interviews for a job. During the important part of the interview, I experienced such radiating pain in my lower abdomen that I had never felt in my entire life. I saw clots of blood gushing out. I was so unprepared for such an eventuality. I rolled up almost a total roll of toilet paper to help get me home to rest. I was alone for the next 3 days resting and not knowing what I had been through. About a year later, I got pregnant, and after about 10 weeks, I miscarried. This experience made me realize what had occurred the year before. The pain and the clots were strikingly similar. So, I knew that experience was a miscarriage. The third time I became pregnant with twins and during the end of first trimester, I miscarried again! The uncertainty of not knowing if we had lost both our babies was hard on my heart. As the pregnancy proceeded with one vanishing twin, we were grateful for our one baby. Multiple hospitalizations, bed rest for almost the entire pregnancy and a cervical surgical procedure to prevent premature labor led to a decision of an elective cesarean at 36 weeks gestation. Throughout my pregnancy and hours of alone time, the holy book of Quran kept constant company giving me solace and strength.

On hindsight, all along this journey of uncertain events, I remember never asking the question, "Why Me?" — NEVER. All my heart knew was 'Just Surrender'.

وَيَمْكُرُونَ وَيَمْكُرُ اللَّهُ وَاللَّهُ خَيْرُ الْمَاكِرِينَ

We plan, and God plans… God is the best of planners.

Giving birth can be an intense and transformative experience and we are biologically wired to experience it. The loss of this physiological experience can be deeply grieving for mind-body and creates a spiritual vacuum leaving our consciousness wounded at multiple levels. The hours, months and many years felt delusional. I had no way to express it — it was *preverbal and primal.*

Prematurity was not an easy state to make sense of for a new first-time mother. After several miscarriages, there was this obsession to be on a hypervigilance state of mind like an animal when she needs to protect her baby from the predator. This hypervigilance was further heightened due to loss of joyful breastfeeding experience. My baby couldn't feed effectively and needed constant body contact to feel safe, to feed and sleep. I battled with alternating feelings of inadequacy, confusion and grief.

237

Even with its best intention, the social and healthcare system fell short of providing the ecosystem required with an abysmal state of denial and no acknowledgement for a new mother to thrive into maternal confidence that becomes the bedrock of the family and social fabric of humanity.

Pain is the window through which God's light enters.

Excruciating pain and the challenges of breastfeeding continued as I frantically looked for help for my frail baby. Each time the baby would breastfeed, I would constantly feel the sense of something crawling in my body. With the writhing pain from frequent — almost every hour of day and night — feedings, I was in constant tears. Over the next two years, even though every feeding was toe curling, my desire continued to nurture my baby at my bosom.

The only constant motivation besides my own family was provided by a German woman who volunteered for an international support group called La Leche League International. Close association with the organization revealed just how many mothers were desperately needing help and the how widespread this need was across the world.

I quickly deepened my connections with professionals across the world and mothers through my accreditation, certification and volunteer work in the field of lactation. Spending vast amounts of time with mothers from various parts of India gave me a very personal feel of the struggle these mothers were going through. It made me connect with the community in a very different way.

At some point during this journey, I recognized that there was a clinical condition called a "tongue tie" that could have been impeding my baby's breastfeeding. Plunging into this subject connected me with a very large network of lactation consultants and other mothers who had come from very similar backgrounds of struggle. I recognized that many of those in this profession came from the heart due to the magnanimity of the struggle. Most were led to this profession.

Healing is not fixing pain it is a spiritual process

The deafening cries of mothers pierced right through my heart. No words, no feelings, no description, no acknowledgment, no comfort can remove the surmountable grief of these mothers at the loss of breastfeeding. Never can we imagine even an ounce of the pain, the loss, the emptiness, the shock and the staggering turn in their lives.

With a tear in my eye, I felt the shame of what humankind has become without a womb of ecosystem to thrive for these mothers. These stories of pain had to be told. How? The answer came from the stillness in my heart that I must 'Create' as many ripples of love, peace and harmony in little ways that I can every day of my life. Sowing that seed is the pursuit and purpose of life and requires me to cleanse myself from inside out. Like a song goes:

"Small acts we do together, even though we are alone, changes the world for the better; so we can call it home."

The breastfeeding challenges were less clinical issues but more of phenomena that had layers of various social issues such as poverty of acknowledgment, rampant dismissal, women's lack of voice, loss of empowerment, gender issues, and the hollowness in the marital relationships.

It was becoming clear to me that this was not so much about "tongue tie" surgery or baby feeding but the underlying issue of dismissal of physical and emotional experiences of women, which is prevalent in all areas of life, including medical and maternal care.

Were we perhaps nurturing a society that sees pain experienced by a woman as 'normal'? In our pursuit to dismiss, do we even forget that all the mother is doing is to protect essential breastfeeding which becomes the fabric of immunity for her developing baby's lifetime?

Do we forget that breastfeeding is a rite of passage for every woman who wishes to breastfeed and has held this baby in her womb for 9 months?

It was never: Why me? But why not me! Pain for me always symbolizes a pivotal energy that gives us an opportunity to dig a grave and bury ourselves or gather our feathers and take a flight!

I wanted to make a film at that point, but I didn't know how because I was not a filmmaker. I felt strongly that something would come to help me through this process. A few years after that, I began supporting a mother who happened to be a documentary filmmaker. She said, "I want to help you."

Seven years down this journey, the documentary film, *Untying Breastfeeding* was finally premiered in Brisbane, Australia. I have a vivid memory of a standing ovation for the film that night and can't even begin to share how I felt at that point, My entire consciousness was healing from all the wounds during pregnancy, birth, and especially the lack of bonding that I had experienced with my baby.

When you share the pain and the deep wounds, they become powerful seeds of change.

I was humbled for the standing ovation for the film that seemed to last forever. The journey of the intent of the film has reached its first wave and I know this will continue to be passed on across the world. Since then, the film has been watched and screened in more than 1,500 cities in the world, in various communities, and to various people, and consistently the response has been exactly the same — overwhelmingly touched.

This led me to seek many other different projects related with the clinical condition of "tongue tie". This condition needed a voice of education in the world and once again I felt called to become that voice. A few changemakers from various countries cofounded the global society: International Consortium of Oral Ankylofrenulae Professionals (ICAP) with a vision to spread the knowledge amongst the clinical community globally via conferences and setting golden standards of care.

This has been my journey. Since its inception, Nourish & Nurture has been engaging in many projects and seeking to bring more synergy and understanding across India and throughout the world. Collaborative efforts with a global institute from Canada to bring high quality lactation education into India and also with ongoing efforts to develop our own local education on breastfeeding became the central vision of Nourish and Nurture Academy & Center of Excellence in Lactation. The larger vision is to ensure that high quality tiered and affordable support is available and provided to every mother and breastfeeding family who seek support. The health care and wellbeing support must follow egalitarianism across various strata of society. The project is already manifesting and it is still miles before we sleep. I am forever grateful for all of the beautiful souls who came into my life to work synergistically to pave this path.

What really drives me is realizing the power of every single conscious soul on this earth. Even if I brought about so much change within myself through this journey in the last 14 years, I can just imagine what it could be like if we could synergize similar heart energies and similar consciousness and stimulate that through our society and community. There's so much good that can be done — so much good. People are waiting to just be supported, to find their own light inside.

How do people walk in the path of life with a sense of clarity, a sense of hope, and the ability to live their truth? If each person begins to live their truth, the world is transformed. The only place that needs healing to change this entire system is birth. If we lose the focus of holding space for the mother and baby during that sacred time of birth and providing that kind of nourishment and care and support and if it requires us to walk a thousand miles, we must do it. If we could heal birth for a safe and supported birth, I think it will transform all the other wounds in this world. Everything is a wound taken away at birth.

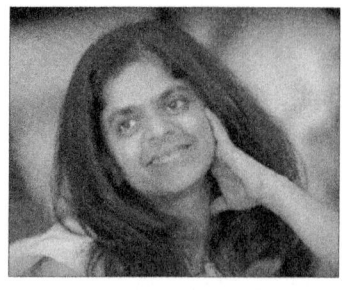

Effath Yasmin is India's leading Biodynamic Craniosacral Therapist, award-winning International Board-Certified Lactation Consultant, Bach Flower Practitioner (Level 2), international speaker and award-winning documentary filmmaker. Her approach stems from the fundamental truth that human organisms are complete and self-regulatory.

Her treatment approach is to support the mind, body, and spirit rather than intervention. Yasmin serves on many international and national boards, has been published in international journals and has spear-headed and dedicated her life to many projects with a central mission of advocacy, education, and awareness for an integrative multidisciplinary wellness approach worldwide. Her international award-winning film, *Untying Breastfeeding*, exposes the glaring unseen obstacles to birth and breastfeeding that can help restore motherhood and has been widely celebrated in 1,500 cities worldwide.

A Call to Action

Birthing The New Humanity – A Global Movement!

We hope these expert stories have inspired you and given you the missing keys to heal yourself, your family, and the planet.

A very real existential crisis is occurring in humanity, one that deserves our attention more than anything else. We balance our innate intelligence with selling our soul and putting false hopes in the power of artificial intelligence.

Just as technology is rapidly changing, so is our collective understanding of human development. Even though contemporary western science is still grappling with the concept of consciousness, no one can deny that we are conscious. Babies in the womb are also conscious; they are actually learning and downloading subconscious programs that will run their lives and consequently our societies and the planet.

Love is our greatest power. It is the very fabric of life. Like the sunrise, emerging from a dark night, love is triumphing and bringing life, nurturing care and wisdom back into our global village. We need to become conscious, loving co-creators of our human family, aware of the awe-inspiring intelligence and beauty of the incarnation process of a soul into human existence.

Birthing The New Humanity is a global community whose mission is to bring the new early parenting, birth, and healing paradigms, infusing them with raised awareness, love, and wisdom, so that our collective dreams come true.

Our vision:
Mothers, once again revered and supported by men, are taking their central place in society. Drying their children's tears, letting them know they are safe and loved unconditionally, they are bringing peace to the world. Fathers are equally respected and honored for their benevolence. Their children enjoy optimum conditions to develop harmoniously, reach their full potential, and be empowered to contribute their unique gifts to the world.

We invite you to participate in making this vision a reality. The co-authors and experts are available on the Birthing The New Humanity (BTNH) app to support you. You may meet them during live events, masterclasses, and courses and continue to learn and benefit from their wisdom and knowledge.

Here are a few action steps you can take:

Download the Birthing The New Humanity app here:

After registering on the app and downloading the FREE gift:

- Test your knowledge with the Womb to Thrive – Missing Keys Quiz
- Discover the authors in the app directory
- Listen to the Womb to Thrive authors' podcast
- Attend the Expert Live Events
- Continue learning and being supported as a BTNH Member
- Take a professional training (e-courses available in 2022)
- Seek support and empowerment to transform early trauma
- Share this book with family, friends, healthcare providers, podcast hosts, media, and your government representatives
- Tell your friends and families that babies are conscious in the womb
- Offer greater consideration for pregnant mothers and fathers
- Prepare in body, mind, and spirit before conceiving a baby
- Support mothers to live healthy, happy, empowered pregnancies
- Use and share the BTNH app to support our movement and raise awareness
- Volunteer to help our community grow and make a greater impact

Professionals:

- List your business, services, and products in the BTNH app directory
- Become a professional member to receive ongoing education and support
- Offer a masterclass and your course through the app
- Become a BTNH mentor
- Apply to be interviewed on the BTNH podcast
- Become a speaker at BTNH summits and events

Organizations:

- Become a BTNH partner
- Invite your members to download the App
- Invite our experts to speak on podcasts, to employees and at events
- Inform employees that pregnant mothers are building our future world
- Improve your organization's support of pregnancy, birth, postnatal care, and breastfeeding
- Always make decisions for the highest good of our global human family

Thank you for your time, attention, and love. We look forward to getting to know you and welcoming you as a co-creator of our thriving global family and planet!

Printed in Great Britain
by Amazon

79267666R00142